# CHAIR YOGA FOR SENIORS OVER 60

## FOR WEIGHT LOSS, BALANCE AND STRENGTH

## DISCLAIMER

This book is intended to provide readers with general information about yoga exercises and routines. The content provided is not a substitute for professional medical advice, diagnosis, or treatment. Engaging in any exercise program carries the risk of injury. While the author and publisher have made every effort to ensure the safety of the exercises and routines described in this book, they cannot guarantee that they are appropriate for every individual. Always seek the advice of a qualified healthcare provider with any questions you may have regarding a medical condition or physical exercise regimen if you are unsure. If you experience pain, dizziness, discomfort, or any other symptoms while performing any of the exercises described in this book, stop immediately and consider seeking medical attention. By voluntarily participating in any of the exercises shown in this publication, you accept the risk of any potential injury.

# 2 BOOKS IN 1

**Congrats on your investment in this book. Inside are 2 books:**

The first one is a Chair Yoga for Weight Loss book. It shows you how to lose weight while building your flexibility and strength.

The 2nd book is for those who are mobility limited or time-scarce and includes safe Chair Yoga exercises that were reviewed to be safe and effective for seniors.

## Secret To Increasing Your Physical Limit As A Senior

As seniors, we have some extra considerations when exercising. Our aging bodies are more prone to injury, and yet, if we never move, our body begins to deteriorate. So how do you balance these 2 conflicting realities? Before any injuries and the effects of immobility and aging, our physical bodies had a high level of discomfort threshold before we reach our physical limits. Once we do, you may experience pain or get overly fatigued:

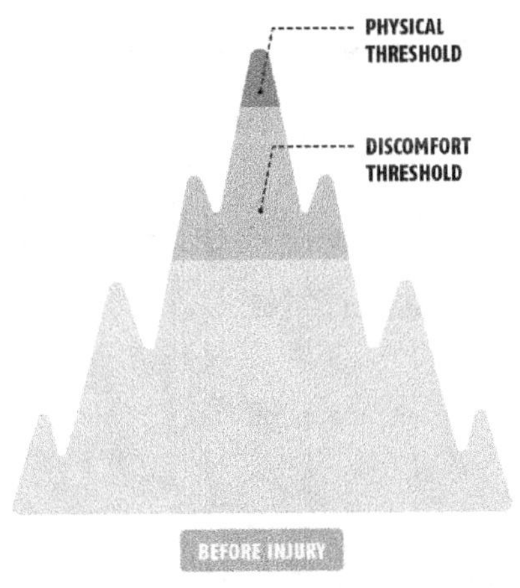


However, as different factors creep into aging, our physical threshold decreases. Aging effects include nutrition, immobility, the natural aging process, osteoporosis, a bad knee, or weight and balance issues, we start to lower our discomfort threshold before we get "inflamed" or "overdo" it. With this lower discomfort threshold, especially with chronic pain, if you over do it, you reach your limits and are out for a few days. With chronic pain patients sometimes you flare up for a few days, or if you're not in chronic pain, you find your muscles super sore and you have trouble moving for the next few days:

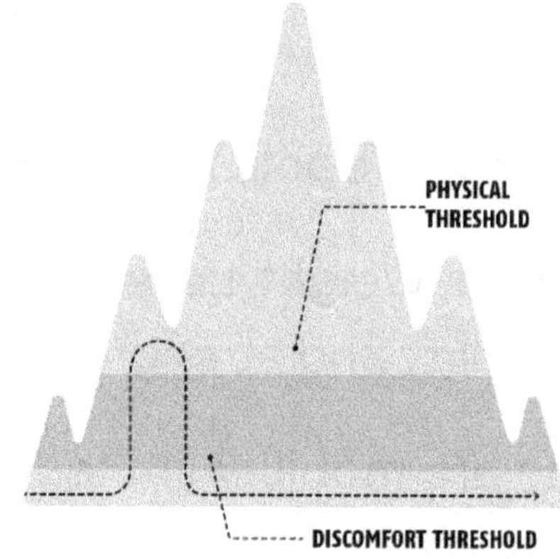


The solution? Pacing. By pacing within our threshold, we avoid the flare ups or over exercising:

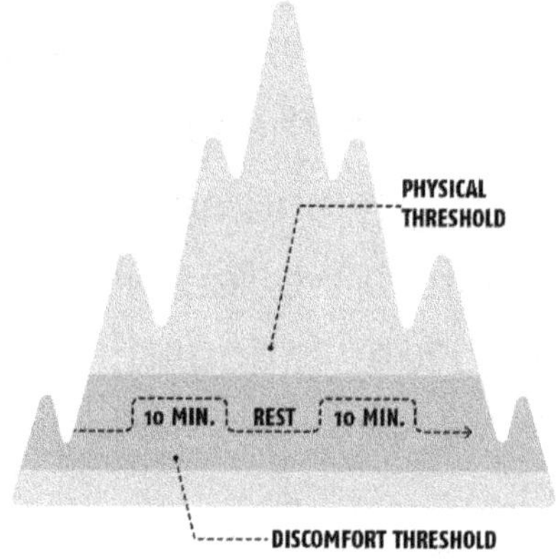


Consistent pacing then starts to increase confident and our new tolerance limits, raising overall conditioning and strength:

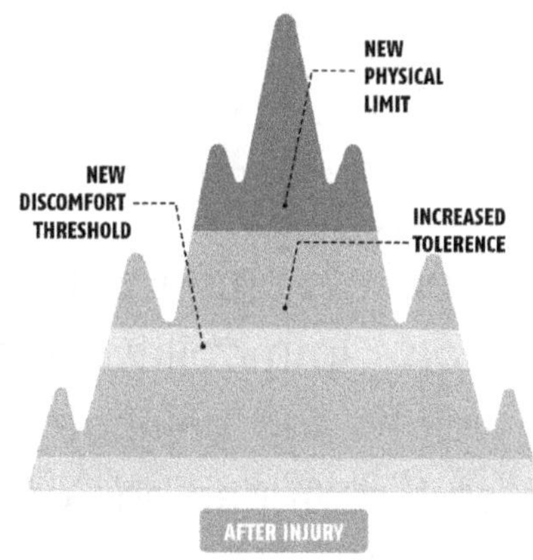

So the answer is to neither push through hard like we did when we were young, nor is it to call it quits and give up. The most effective strategy is to slowly increase the amount of time spent in gentle movement and exercise, and aim to slowly increase your baseline into a level of activity that you love.

So, instead of constantly pushing and running into injuries or inflammation, we gradually pace the exercises to your current comfort. The key is small consistency. With consistently, pretty quickly you realize your previous threshold has increased and you just get better and better from there.

So, go at your own pace, but be consistent. Paradoxically, being aware of your limits is the key to surpassing your limits. Go slow by selecting 10 exercises when you first start and try them out for a week. Don't try to do everything at once. As you get stronger and more flexible, you can try the workout routines in one of the pages.

## Secret of Trigger Points

While everyone's body is different, one issue for sore muscles or immobility is due to trigger points. While everyone's body is different, I discovered that my chronic pain and immobility issues were coming from weak muscles riddled with trigger points (TrPs). Trigger points are taut muscle bands that have been created that restrict movement and blood flow. If you feel like you have TrPs, a great place to start is Clair Davies's book *The Trigger Point Therapy Workbook.*

So, if you have muscles ridden with TrPs like I did, you must first get rid of those TrPs. But what comes later is a weak TrPs-free muscle. This is where these exercises comes in. After being TrP free, you can use this book to train weak muscles to get stronger since it can work all the slow- and fast-twitch muscle fibers and regulate smaller muscles that aren't stimulated to the same extent by conventional exercises.

Lastly, if you have any questions, you can email me at wall.pilates2@gmail.com.


Love,

-Luna Light

Congrats! Your new book comes with video lessons included. A lot of time and effort went into making this the best exercise book and that applies to our videos too. Completed by a certified Pilates instructor, the moves in the videos are correctly done and easy to follow. Unlike our competitors, you won't have to worry about risking injury, following bad instructions or using improper or dangerous movements.

### HOW TO DOWNLOAD YOUR BONUS VIDEOS:

Write an email to: wall.pilates2@gmail.com

And put **"Senior 60 Chair Yoga"** in the subject line

We will reply promptly (usually within a few hours) so be sure to write the correct email.

# CHAIR YOGA
## FOR WEIGHT LOSS

*Lose Weight and Gain Better Balance,
Posture, Mobility, Strength, and Flexibility*

# Contents

# Introduction

*"Strength does not come from the body. It comes from the will."*
—Mahatma Gandhi

Five years ago, my life took a sudden, unexpected turn. As a personal trainer and former athlete, I was the human version of the Energizer Bunny—running, cycling, and working out in the gym daily.

Then, one beautiful sunny morning, I was on my way to a personal training client's home when a drunk driver smashed into my car.

The accident left me in so much pain that I couldn't walk. My life was now confined to a tiny bedroom at a friend's house, lying in a bed staring at the ceiling and feeling sorry for myself.

Hi, my name is Luna, and strangely, that accident opened up a whole new world of opportunity for me.

It didn't happen right away. Like anyone in this situation, I experienced all the emotions of recovery—denial, anger, acceptance, sadness, and loss. All I could think about in the dark weeks after the accident was what I was no longer able to do.

Finally, I realized that I needed to start taking control of my situation. Rather than fixating on what I couldn't do, I began looking for exercises that I could accomplish.

After a few weeks, I could sit up in a chair. I then began to discover low-impact forms of exercise that would allow me to regain my strength, muscle tone, and flexibility. I learned about yoga, Pilates, and somatic movements.

I slowly began to find pain relief and regain my strength through these methods. But there was still one problem: weight gain!

The sudden transition from a highly active to a sedentary lifestyle added pounds to my hips, butt, and thighs. I'd always relied on running-type exercises for weight loss, so at first, I didn't know where to turn—stuck as I was in my chair.

That was when I discovered chair yoga for weight loss.

At first, I was doubtful. How could I lose weight sitting on my butt? But as I researched and then applied what I was learning, I discovered that chair yoga was, indeed, an effective means of weight loss for mobility-challenged people. And the results on my body were undeniable.

Through a combination of chair yoga and mindful eating, I was able to drop the extra pounds I'd piled on while also improving my strength and flexibility. Even my posture improved!

I've now become a passionate advocate of exercise for people with mobility challenges. Over the past five years, I've met hundreds of wonderful people frustrated that their mobility limitations prevented them from doing weight loss exercises. Maybe you're feeling that way, too.

Or maybe you're a person who just doesn't have the time or circumstances to do conventional exercise to keep the pounds off. Chair yoga exercises for weight loss are ideal for you, too. In fact, you can do them right at your computer, seamlessly incorporating these gentle yet effective movements into your daily routine.

I'm excited to open up the world of chair yoga for weight loss to you in the pages of this guidebook. Here's a form of exercise that meets you where you are, allowing you to achieve your weight loss goals safely and effectively. And it only takes fifteen minutes to twenty minutes daily.

Are you ready to embrace the transformative power of chair yoga for weight loss?

Let's do it together.

Love, Luna.

# Who This Book Is For

If you want to lose weight safely and effectively without putting impact stress on your joints, then this book is for you. As a former athlete, I know firsthand that these exercises can benefit both able-bodied and mobility-limited people on their weight loss journey.

## People with Mobility Issues

People with mobility issues will especially benefit from this guide. Traditional weight loss workouts are very lower-body focused. Whether running, jumping, cycling, or stepping, they require you to propel your body forward to burn calories. People with mobility issues are excluded from many of these activities.

*Chair Yoga for Weight Loss* fills a gaping hole in the weight loss exercise market for people with mobility issues. It provides accessible movements that, when done in the manner prescribed, will bring real results.

## People with Health Issues

People with health issues, such as arthritis, chronic pain, mobility limitations, or cardiovascular conditions, will also benefit greatly from *Chair Yoga for Weight Loss*. These movements are gentle, soothing, and progressive. They will provide your body with the stress it needs to adapt, but they will do so in a way that meets you where you are in terms of physical health.

## Seniors

Seniors will especially benefit from *Chair Yoga for Weight Loss*. These exercises are designed to accommodate the balance and mobility issues that many older folks experience.

I work with a lot of people who have gained weight since retiring. Issues like arthritis often prevent them from running or sometimes even walking for weight loss. Yet chair yoga combined with healthy eating has helped all of them to drop the pounds and reclaim their vitality.

## Time-Poor and Deskbound People

If you're a person who knows they should be exercising for weight loss but just can't find the time or simply doesn't know how to start, *Chair Yoga for Weight Loss* is for you, too. The exercises are especially beneficial for people who spend long hours at the computer.

# **How to Use** This Book

As a personal fitness trainer, I love to work one-on-one with people who want to improve their fitness, lose weight, and become a better version of themselves. My goal in writing this book has been to make you feel as if I'm right alongside you, guiding you as you become increasingly confident with chair yoga exercises for weight loss.

As a result, I've made this guide as user-friendly as I know how. There are two main sections:

- Essential Knowledge
- The Exercises

In the Essential Knowledge section, you'll discover why chair yoga is an effective weight loss tool and how to incorporate it into your lifestyle. I'll also provide some vital guidance on blood flow, muscle movement, and how to breathe during exercise.

This section also makes sense of the confusing topic of how to eat for successful weight loss. I'll cut through all the white noise to provide you with six science-based eating habits that really work for long-term fat loss.

While you may be tempted to jump directly to the Exercise section of the book, please take the time to absorb the Essential Knowledge section first. It's packed with tips and information to make your weight loss journey smoother and more successful.

The Exercise section has four parts, summarized by the acronym WAGU. I'm not talking about premium Japanese beef but rather a 4-step exercise routine that's safe and effective:

1. **Warm Up:** These gentle movements will activate your muscles, get the blood flowing, and promote joint lubrication.

2. **Awareness in Movement:**  These exercises increase the intensity and range of the exercises, placing more stress on your muscles and getting your heart rate up slightly.
3. **Gain Gentle Momentum:** These moves are designed to increase your heart rate as they engage specific muscles through a full range of movement.
4. **Unwinding Relaxation:** These cool-down exercises are designed to return your body to its relaxed, pre-exercise state.

I encourage you to follow the WAGU sequence as you perform the exercises. Begin by selecting five moves from the Warmup section. Choose a range of exercises to warm both the upper and lower body.

Next, select four moves from the Awareness in Movement section. Again, choose a range of moves to engage all your body's muscles.

Choose four more exercises from the Awareness in Movement section. These exercises should be done faster than the previous ones and should get you puffing slightly.

Finish your workout by selecting five moves from the Unwinding section.

# ESSENTIAL KNOWLEDGE

# **Why Chair** Yoga?

*"Yoga is not about touching your toes. It's about what you learn on the way down."*
*—Jigar Gor*

Chair yoga offers a safe and accessible form of exercise for everybody. The use of a chair as a prop offers stability and support, reducing the risk of injuries commonly associated with traditional exercises. This makes it ideal for seniors, people undergoing rehab, and folks with mobility issues who may be prone to balance challenges or joint discomfort.

Chair yoga increases strength and mobility. The gentle movements and poses allow you to gradually build muscle strength and improve flexibility without putting undue stress on your joints. The stabilizing force of the chair enables users to engage in a full range of motion, promoting better circulation and overall physical well-being.

The convenience of chair yoga is a huge bonus. The ability to exercise while seated makes it an accessible option for those who may struggle to find time for more traditional forms of exercise.

The versatility of chair yoga allows it to be combined with other fitness activities or pursued as a standalone practice, providing flexibility for different preferences and schedules.

Chair yoga is also an extremely cost-effective solution. It can be performed with just a chair and a minimum of space.

# **Using Chair Yoga** for Weight Loss

*"Yoga means addition – addition of energy, strength, and beauty to body, mind, and soul."*
—Amit Ray

People with mobility issues often feel helpless when it comes to losing weight. They know they've got to exercise, but their limitations stop them from doing what most experts advise for weight loss.

Chair yoga is the solution to that dilemma. It provides a form of weight loss exercise that is low-impact and accessible, strengthens your muscles, and improves your flexibility as it burns off those extra calories.

But let's not kid ourselves here. You will not burn as many calories in a fifteen-minute chair yoga workout as you would running on a treadmill or exercising on a stair stepper. That is why we need to get serious about the other side of the weight loss equation—nutrition.

Weight maintenance is essentially a matter of caloric balance. To lose weight, you have to create a negative calorie balance. That means that you burn more calories for energy than you take in through food. This forces your body to draw upon its stored calories in the form of body fat to make up the difference.

The more days you can do that, the more body fat you will lose. It is the combination of a balanced diet and exercise that will bring you success.

# **Chair Yoga** Essential Equipment

*"Yoga is the journey of the self, through the self, to the self."*
—The Bhagavad Gita

The following essential equipment will help to keep your chair yoga workouts safe, comfortable, and effective:

## A Sturdy Chair

Your chair should have four sturdy legs and a back support. Chairs with armrests will also provide enhanced support to keep you upright, especially when doing lower-body exercises.

Avoid chairs that are overly bulky and hard to move. It needs to provide solid, rigid support when you are leaning on it. This rules out our rocking chairs and chairs with wheels or rollers.

Ideally, your selected chair should provide decent padding to keep you comfortable. You may choose to sit on a pillow for extra comfort.

## Footwear

Many people prefer to do their chair yoga workout in bare feet. This enhances their sensory experience and provides a sense of freedom. If you would rather wear shoes, make sure that they are comfortable and have nonslip soles.

## Clothing

Your workout attire should be comfortable and form-fitting. Do not wear tight clothing that may restrict your range of movement or cut off your circulation. On the other hand, you don't want your clothing to be so loose that it gets caught up when you are exercising.



Fill a water bottle with fresh H2O and place it alongside your chair. Sup from it between exercises to keep yourself well hydrated.



There should be at least a meter (3'3") of clear space around your chair. This will ensure that you have an unrestricted range of movement.

# Six Weight Loss Nutrition Habits

*"Exercise is king, nutrition is Queen, put them together, and you've got a kingdom."*
—Jack Lalanne

Nutrition is the key to weight loss. The problem is that there's so much confusion about how to do it that many people simply throw up their hands in frustration and return to how they've always eaten.

What's needed is some simple, straightforward direction that actually works.

Now, let me make it clear that I'm not a nutritionist. However, as a personal trainer, I have recommended six simple nutrition habits to help hundreds of people lose weight over the years. These habits, combined with exercise, have helped my clients achieve their weight loss goals healthily and sustainably.

Let's check them out:

We've already discussed the importance of maintaining a negative calorie balance, where your body uses up more energy than it takes in. There are several ways to do this.

A common method is to work out how many calories your body needs to consume to supply your energy needs and then count calories each day to ensure that you are under that number.

I can tell you through experience with my clients that this is not a sustainable method. Counting calories with every meal is simply too time-consuming, even when using weight loss apps like MyFitnessPal.

A far more practical and effective method is intermittent fasting. It's a method that I personally use and recommend to my clients. Here's what it involves:

1. On Sunday, complete your last meal of the day by 7 p.m.

2. Do not eat again until 11 a.m. on Monday.

3. Eat three meals, spread 2.5–3 hours apart between 11 a.m. and 7 p.m.

4. Continue this pattern Monday through Friday.

5. From Friday at 7 a.m. until Sunday at 7 p.m., there are no restrictions on when you eat.

Here's why this form of intermittent fasting is so effective:

- It allows you to achieve a negative calorie balance without counting calories.

- It depletes your muscle cells of glucose, the body's primary energy source. This forces the body to turn to its backup energy source—stored body fat.

- It increases energy and promotes the release of hormones such as growth hormone and testosterone.

- It increases insulin sensitivity, helping the body better regulate blood glucose levels. Improved insulin sensitivity contributes to weight management by reducing the likelihood of excess glucose being stored as fat.

## Habit #2: Eat Protein with Every Meal

Protein is the building material of your body. It helps to maintain muscle mass while also burning off body fat due to its denseness and higher thermic effect. Protein is also very filling, helping to prevent grazing and snacking between meals.

I recommend having a palm-sized serving of protein with every meal. Include organic eggs, chicken, and fish sources for the best quality complete proteins (a protein that contains all nine essential amino acids).

## Habit #3: Eat Vegetables or Fruits with Every Meal

Plants contain vitamins, minerals, and essential phytochemicals for optimal physiological functioning. They also help balance your pH levels and provide much-needed fiber for enhanced digestion.

Fiber-rich plant-based foods help keep you full so that you consume fewer calories. I recommend keeping the fruit bowl on your kitchen bench stocked with various attractive-looking fruits. Develop the habit of reaching for an apple, banana, or orange when you feel peckish between meals.

Include two to three servings of vegetables with your dinner meal. Strive for variety, including choices like leafy greens, colorful bell peppers, broccoli, cauliflower, carrots, and tomatoes. These vegetables provide essential vitamins and minerals and offer a diverse range of antioxidants that support overall health.

The healthiest way to cook vegetables is through methods such as steaming, roasting, or sautéing with minimal oil. These cooking techniques help preserve the nutritional value of the vegetables while enhancing their natural flavors.

Avoid overcooking, as this can lead to nutrient loss. Experiment with herbs and spices to add flavor without relying on excessive salt or unhealthy sauces.

Most of your carbohydrates should come from vegetables and fruits. Avoid processed foods high in sugar, as these will cause insulin spikes, leading to increased fat storage and energy crashes.

Here are half a dozen processed carb foods to avoid, along with healthy replacement suggestions:

**1. Sugary Breakfast Cereals:**

Replace with steel-cut oats or quinoa porridge topped with fresh berries and a sprinkle of nuts. This provides a fiber-rich, satisfying breakfast without the added sugars.

**2. White Bread:**

Replace with: Whole grain or sprouted grain bread which contains more fiber and nutrients. Alternatively, try lettuce wraps for a low-carb option.

**3. Sugary Drinks:**

Replace with: Water, herbal tea, or infused water with slices of citrus, cucumber, or mint. Sugary drinks contribute empty calories and can lead to rapid blood sugar spikes.

**4. Flavored Yogurt with Added Sugars:**

Replace with: Greek yogurt or plain yogurt with fresh fruit and a drizzle of honey or a sprinkle of cinnamon. This reduces added sugars while increasing protein and beneficial probiotics.

**5. Packaged Snack Bars:**

Replace with: Homemade energy bars using oats, nuts, seeds, and dried fruit. This allows you to control the ingredients and avoid hidden sugars.

**6. Potato Chips and Other Processed Snacks:**

Replace with: Air-popped popcorn seasoned with herbs or a handful of mixed nuts for a satisfying crunch without the unhealthy additives. These options provide healthier fats and more nutrients.

## Habit #5: Eat Healthy Fats Every Day

Add healthy fats to your diet in the form of avocados, nuts, extra virgin olive oil, and fish oil supplements. These are very calorie-dense, helping you feel fuller faster. Healthy fats provide a sustained energy source while stabilizing blood sugar levels to prevent cravings.

## Habit #6: Drink More Water

Sixty percent of your body is water. It's essential for life and well-being. Yet, 80 percent of Americans don't drink enough of it, with a large proportion of them walking around in a state of dehydration.

Among its many other health benefits, water promotes weight loss. People often mistake thirst for hunger. So, getting into the habit of drinking a glass of water before a meal will help to moderate your calorie intake.

Drinking water also increases your metabolic rate. Drinking half a gallon of water daily (about two liters) will increase your energy burn by around ninety-three calories.

# **Luna's Insights** on Weight Loss

**_"Don't dig your grave with your own knife and fork."_**
_—Old English Proverb_

Despite all the marketing hype, there is no magic pill for fat loss. The real key to fat loss is to adopt the underlying principle of establishing a caloric deficit.

When you are in a calorie deficit, you will lose weight, regardless of what else you do. However, you won't start seeing results for a few weeks. That means you must be patient, especially in the early days. Avoid the temptation to jump on the scales every day/week—feel it in the fit of your clothing and your newfound energy.

Take it slowly. Introduce new habits that work for you and maintain your workout consistency. The longer you do this, the better results you will get.

Don't allow yourself to latch onto the excuse that you don't have time to make healthy meals or that you're adjusting to eating like everyone else in the family. Those excuses don't cut it anymore—not with all the healthy meal options available these days.

## Weight Loss Is Not Fat Loss

You may have noticed that I refer to fat loss rather than weight loss. That's because there is a big difference between the two. Unless you appreciate that difference, you will forever be spinning your fat loss wheels.

For over a century, we've been sold on the fallacy that your diminishing weight on the scale is your sure sign of success. Just think of shows like _The Biggest Loser_. Nothing else matters but getting that scale down.

The truth is that you should never be interested in losing pure weight. Being obsessed with bringing your weight down on the scale is dumb—pure and simple.

The bathroom scale cannot differentiate between muscle and fat. Nor can it tell if you are losing water or vital minerals. All it can tell you is that your body weight has decreased. That in itself is a useless piece of information.

You never want to lose muscle. Yet, that is exactly what you are losing on most extreme calorie-restricted diets. Muscle is a lot denser than fat. So when a person's body goes into starvation because they have severely cut back their caloric intake, it turns to its muscle stores and catabolizes itself.

When you step on the scale, you feel elated. The scale has come down. But what have you actually done to your body?

You have robbed it of its body shaping, firming, strength-enhancing muscle mass. Meanwhile, all your fat is still there where it's always been.

Extreme calorie reduction diets will also squeeze water weight from your body, especially in the initial stages. We've already discussed the vital importance of water in the body, so you know that is not a good thing. Yet again, it fools people into thinking they are losing body fat.

Rather than relying on the scale to gauge your weight loss, use the mirror, the tape measure, and your body fat percentage. You can buy electronic scales that measure your body fat level for not much more than a standard set of scales.

## A Powerful Tool to Control Your Food Intake

After working with hundreds of weight loss clients, I have found that a significant step to weight loss involves …

*Learning to eat as a response to genuinely feeling hungry rather than as an emotional response to what's going on in your life.*

A super effective tool I use with my clients to do this is the Hunger Gauge.

The Hunger Gauge has six levels:

1. You are desperately hungry and experiencing clear signs of hunger, such as feeling shaky or faint.

2. You are very hungry; your stomach is rumbling, and you feel slightly tired.

3. You are moderately hungry; you have an appetite for food and a pleasant sense of anticipation.

4. You feel satisfied. You could be tempted to eat dessert, but it is not essential.

5. You are too full; you left it a little late to stop eating because you couldn't resist the temptation of another small helping.

6. You are very full; you ignored all the signs to stop eating and now feel weighed down. You may also experience indigestion and heartburn.

You should eat when you are at Level 3 on the Hunger Gauge. Stop when you reach Level 4.

Whenever you feel tempted to eat, go back to the Hunger Gauge and analyze where you are. If it's not Level 3, don't eat!

# **Mobility, Flexibility,** Balance, & Posture

*"Embrace the power of movement, for in the dance of flexibility and mobility, you discover the freedom to explore life's boundless possibilities."*
*—Maya Taylor*

Mobility, flexibility, balance, and posture are all needed for functional, pain-free movement. Chair yoga improves each of these areas. Here's an overview:

## Mobility

Mobility is strength through the full range of motion of an exercise. Unlike flexibility, it relies on the muscle alone to produce the range of movement. So, a flexible person may be able to raise their straightened leg quite high with the assistance of their arm. A mobile person, however, will be able to manipulate their leg or other muscles without any help at all.

Many people focusing exclusively on strength training are strong through a limited range of a muscle's motion. Others are very mobile in parts of the body but not in others. We can think of cyclists with well-developed and mobile legs but poor development and mobility in the upper body.

The chair yoga exercises in this book are designed to enhance mobility by engaging various muscle groups and promoting flexibility throughout the entire body. These chair yoga exercises aim to improve joint health and muscle function by incorporating gentle movements and stretches while seated. The emphasis is on cultivating strength within specific muscle ranges and across the complete spectrum of motion.

## Flexibility

Flexibility is the capacity of muscles and joints to stretch easily, allowing for a broader range of motion. Chair yoga improves flexibility through gentle stretches that target key muscle groups. This promotes elongation while also releasing tension. As the days and weeks go by, you will experience greater joint flexibility, allowing you to move more freely.

## Balance

Balance is the ability to maintain control and stability during movements or while stationary. Chair yoga promotes balance through specific poses and exercises that focus on stability. Performing controlled movements and poses while seated strengthens the core muscles and improves proprioception. As a result, you'll be more confident on your feet.

Posture refers to the position of the body while sitting, standing, or moving. Chair yoga exercises emphasize spinal alignment, core engagement, and muscle strengthening to promote an upright and balanced posture. The exercises in this book will also help you become more mindful of your body positioning, reducing strain on the spine and supporting a healthier posture.

# **How to** Breathe

*"Breathe deeply, for with each breath, you inhale the strength to face challenges and exhale the power to let go. In the rhythm of your breath, find the serenity that carries you forward."*
—*Amit Ray*

Breathing is something we've all been doing since the moment we entered this world. So, you'd think that we'd have learned to do it right. The reality is that while we can all breathe to preserve our lives, there are many ways to improve our breathing, especially when paired with exercise.

Deep nasal breathing is the most effective way to breathe in order to produce a relaxed, calm state and energize your body. When you draw in air through the nasal passage, you are able to achieve a greater intake of oxygen to the bloodstream.

Your breathing rate will naturally slow down when you breathe through the nose, producing a calmer state. As a result, your mind will start to relax. It's as if a switch is triggered to counter stress.

## How to Do It

Stand or sit comfortably. Take in a long, deep breath through your nose until the lungs are completely full and your chest is inflated. Breathe deeply, expanding your ribcage outward and allowing the lungs to fill with air. Exhale through pursed lips as if blowing through a straw, engaging your core muscles. Experience the sensation of an abdominal contraction.

Allow the breath to leave your body, exhaling through the mouth slowly. Think about expanding and compressing the diaphragm as if it were an accordion on every inward and outward breath.

## Nasal Breathing Exercise

Do this first thing in the morning upon waking and again in the mid-afternoon (it will provide a caffeine-free way of overcoming the 3 o'clock slump!).

**Step One:** Get comfortable, either standing or sitting.

**Step Two:** Breathe in through the nose for five seconds. Feel your stomach pushing out as the energy giving oxygen fills your lungs.

**Step Three:** Hold for twenty seconds. Feel the oxygen circulating around your body as it gives life to your trillions of cells.

**Step Four:** Repeat this process four more times.

Note: When performing lung exercises, focusing on inflating the lungs upward and outward rather than downward is important. Imagine that the oxygen intake is about to lift you up and carry you skyward.

## The 4-7-8 Breathing Technique

The 4-7-8 breathing technique, developed by Dr. Andrew Weil, promotes calmness and tranquillity. Here's how to do it:

1. Inhale through the nose for four counts.

2. Hold for a count of seven.

3. Exhale audibly for a count of eight, producing a whooshing sound as you do so.

4. Complete four cycles to calm the nervous system post-workout or during stressful moments.

## Box Breathing

Box breathing, which a former navy seal devised, is a fantastic post-workout technique to allow your body to relax and recuperate.

Box breathing involves four steps, each of which is held to a count of four:

(1) Exhale to a count of four.

(2) Wait for a count of four (empty lungs).

(3) Inhale to a count of four.

(4) Hold the air in your lungs for a count of four.

Begin with one to three minutes of continuous box breathing. Then work up to ten minutes per day. Do your box breathing exercises within the hour after your workout.

# The **Story of** Yoga

*"In the attitude of silence the soul finds the path in a clearer light, and what is elusive and deceptive resolves itself into crystal clearness"*
—*Mahatma Gandhi*

The ancient practice of yoga traces its origins back to the spiritual traditions of ancient India. Over the centuries, it has evolved into a holistic system encompassing physical, mental, and spiritual well-being.

Today, yoga, in its many forms, is highly valued as a form of exercise that promotes vitality, strength, and mobility while also reducing stress and encouraging mindfulness.

At its core, yoga is more than just a series of physical postures; it is a philosophy that embraces the union of mind, body, and spirit. The Sanskrit word "yoga" itself translates to "union" or "to yoke," signifying the connection between these essential elements of the human experience.

The journey of yoga involves physical postures (asanas), breath control (pranayama), meditation, and ethical principles that guide practitioners toward a more conscious and intentional way of living.

**Congrats! Your book comes with a bonus: *The Ultimate Kegels Guide.***

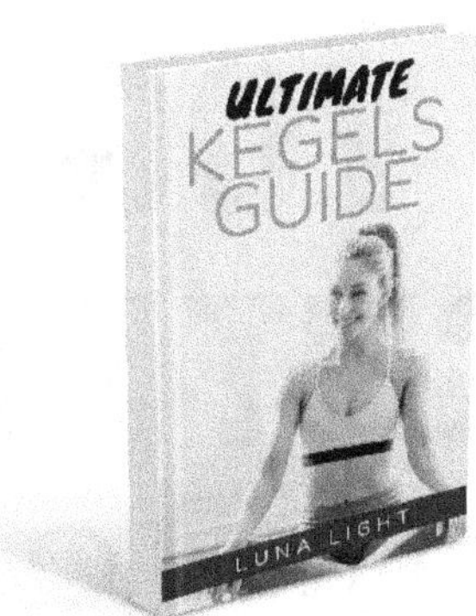

You may have heard of Kegels before... but unfortunately, there is widespread misinformation about hold time, number of repetitions, and how to actually perform the contractions that do more harm than good.

When done right, Kegels are a powerful way to build endurance, increase strength in your core, and enhance your sex life. The Kegels exercise we created comes directly from Tim Sawyer, a top physical therapist who worked with doctors at Stanford University* to develop rehabilitation programs.

This exact Kegels exercise has helped tremendously in improving my pelvic floor tone, enhancing my sex life, and developing a strong core.

All you have to do is go to wallpilates.org to download it for free. Alternatively, scan the QR code below:

---

*    Dr. Wise and Dr. Anderson authored A Headache in the Pelvis: A New Understanding and Treatment for Chronic Pelvic Pain Syndromes and consulted Tim as the main physical therapist for their treatments.

# CHAIR YOGA FOR WEIGHT LOSS
## EXERCISES

# Your **28 Day** Plan

Your chair yoga weight loss plan is very simple. Try out all the movements and pick your favourite for the first 14 days.

- Pick and do 4 Warmup Exercises.

- Pick and do 5 Awareness in Movement Exercises

- Pick and do 5 Gentle Momentum Exercises

- Pick and do 5 Unwinding Relaxation Exercises

For the next 14 days, pick new exercises from the 4 workout groups:

- Pick and do 4 new Warmup Exercises.

- Pick and do 5 new Awareness in Movement Exercises

- Pick and do 5 new Gentle Momentum Exercises

- Pick and do 5 new Unwinding Relaxation Exercises

After the first 28 days, you can try doing all the exercises in this book in one 45 min session. Be sure to rest and recovery whenever you feel at your limit. This is not a race. The movements should feel relaxing and fun.

# WARM-UP EXERCISES

The gentle movements in this section are designed to "wake up" your muscles, moving them through a full range of motion while increasing blood flow and lubricating your joints.

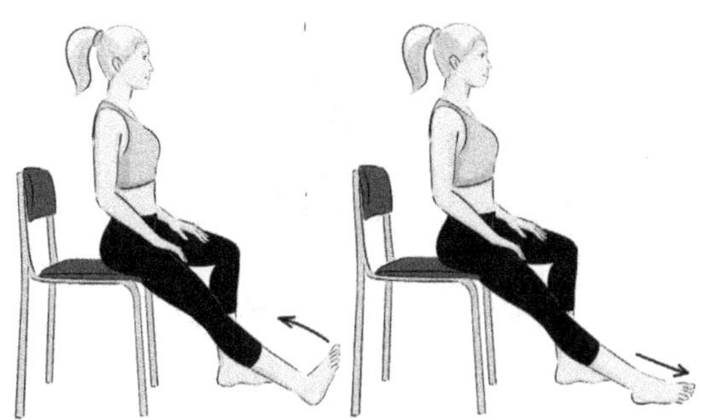

1  Begin by sitting comfortably on a stable chair with your feet flat on the floor and your back straight.

2  Extend one leg forward while keeping the other foot flat on the floor. Point your toes upward, engaging the muscles in your calf and ankle.

3  Begin making slow, controlled circles with your extended ankle in a clockwise direction. Focus on the full range of motion, moving from the toes to the heel. Perform eight to ten circles.

4  Change the direction of the ankle circles to counterclockwise. Again, pay attention to the smooth and controlled movement. Perform eight to ten circles.

5  Repeat on the other leg.

**Tips:**

Ensure that all movements are deliberate and controlled. Avoid jerky or rapid motions, as this warmup is designed to gently increase blood flow and flexibility in the ankle joints.

# Gentle Neck Stretch

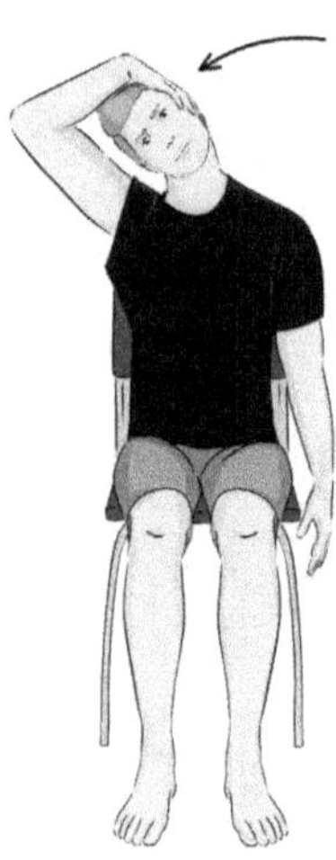

1  Sit tall with your spine erect and your feet flat on the floor. Rest your hands on your thighs or in your lap.

2  Allow your shoulders to relax down away from your ears. Feel the natural lengthening of your spine.

3  Place your right hand on your head with your fingers just above your left ear. Slowly tilt your head to the right, bringing your ear toward your shoulder. Apply gentle pressure with your hand.

4  Avoid lifting or lowering the shoulder; focus on the gentle stretch along the side of your neck.

5  Hold the position for fifteen seconds, feeling a comfortable stretch. You should feel a gentle pull along the opposite side of your neck.

6  Slowly bring your head back to the center, maintaining an upright posture. Do this for five reps.

7  Repeat on the opposite side.

**Tips:**

Avoid sudden or jerky movements to prevent strain. Smooth, deliberate stretches are more effective for releasing tension.

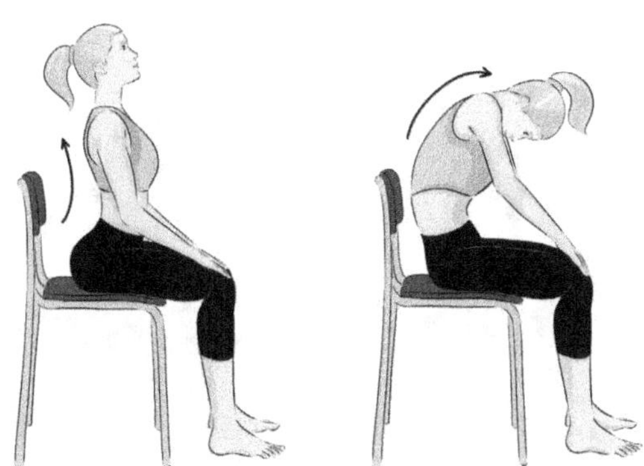

1. Sit on a chair with your feet flat on the floor and your back straight. Place your hands on your knees or thighs.

2. Inhale and arch your back, lifting your chest (cow pose).

3. As you exhale, round your back, tuck your chin to your chest, and draw your navel in (cat pose).

4. Continue to flow between cow and cat poses with your breath, inhaling for the cow and exhaling for the cat.

5. Perform this gentle movement for ten reps, feeling the stretch and release in your spine.

**Tips:**

- You can place your hands on the sides of the chair or hold the armrests for support.

- Keep your movements smooth and controlled, focusing on your breath and the sensations in your back.

# Chair Shoulder Rolls

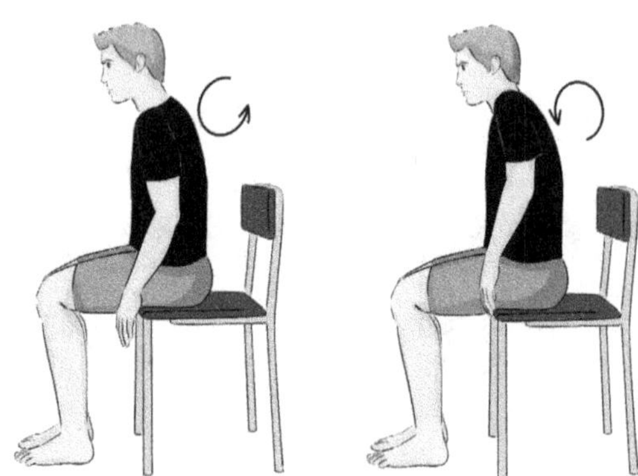

1  Sit with your feet flat on the floor. Ensure your back is straight and your hands are resting on your thighs or in your lap.

2  Allow your shoulders to relax down, away from your ears. Find a neutral position where your spine is aligned and there's no unnecessary tension in the shoulders.

3  Inhale deeply as you lift both shoulders toward your ears in a smooth, circular motion. Exhale as you roll your shoulders forward, bringing them down and around in a circular motion. Complete this forward-rolling motion for ten to fifteen repetitions.

**Tips:**

As you roll your shoulders, focus on the movement of your shoulder blades. Feel them glide along your back during both forward and backward rolls.

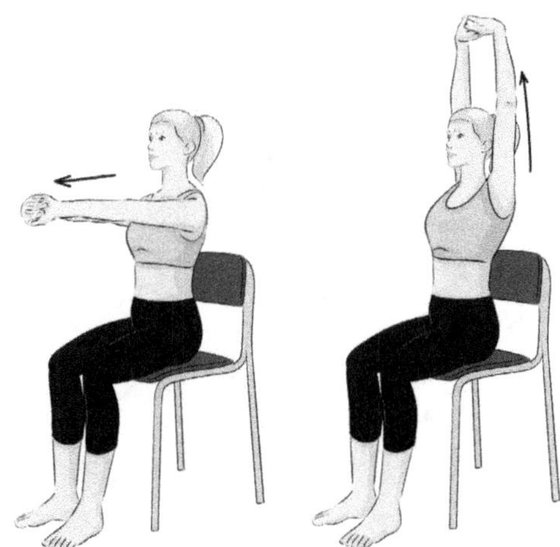

1 Sit upright with an erect spine, and your hands are resting in your lap.

2 Inhale deeply as you extend both arms forward, reaching them overhead. Interlace your fingers in the overhead position.

3 As you extend your arms, lengthen your spine by reaching upward through the fingertips. Feel a gentle stretch along the sides of your body.

4 Hold the overhead position for fifteen seconds, maintaining steady breathing. Focus on elongating your spine and opening up your chest.

5 Exhale as you slowly bring your arms down, returning them to the starting position.

6 Do this exercise for ten reps.

**Tips:**

Gradual Progression: If you're new to stretching, start with a partial overhead reach and gradually progress to a fuller stretch as your flexibility improves. Listen to your body and avoid pushing yourself into discomfort.

# Pike Pulse

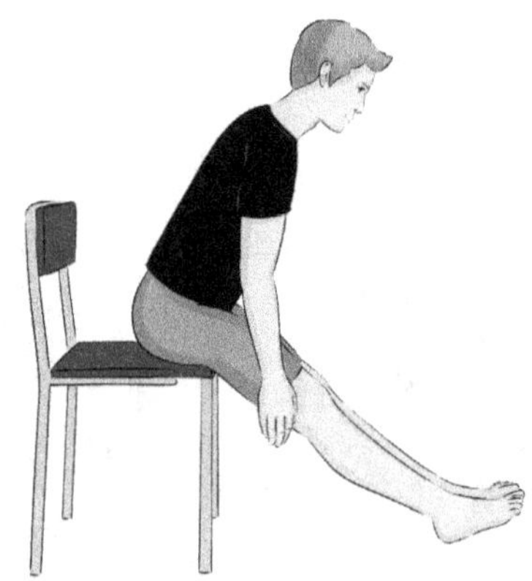

1. Sit on the edge of a sturdy chair with your feet extended in front of you. Ensure your back is straight and your hands are resting on your thighs or in your lap.

2. Activate your core muscles by drawing your navel toward your spine.

3. Inhale as you extend both arms forward at shoulder height, parallel to the floor. Keep your palms facing each other, creating a straight line from your fingertips through your spine.

4. Exhale and hinge at the hips, leaning forward with a straight back. Maintain the engagement in your core to support the movement.

5. Pulse Forward: Once you reach the maximum comfortable stretch forward, initiate small pulsing movements by contracting and releasing your core muscles. Pulse for ten to fifteen repetitions, maintaining control and a steady pace.

6. Inhale as you return to an upright seated position.

**Tips:**

Avoid using momentum and concentrate on engaging your core muscles to guide the pulses.

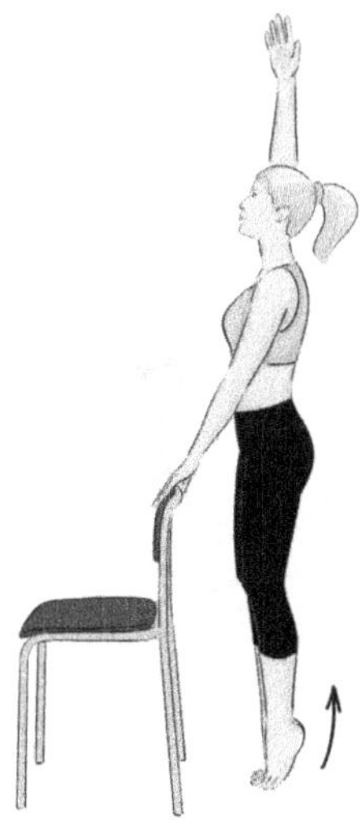

1. Position a sturdy chair in front of you, ensuring it's on a stable surface. Stand with your feet hip-width apart and place your hands on the backrest of the chair for support.

2. Activate your core by drawing your navel toward your spine. This engagement provides stability as you perform the exercise.

3. Rise up on your toes as you raise your right hand overhand and stretch toward the ceiling.

4. Hold the extended position for a five-second count and release.

5. Repeat on the other side.

6. Do this exercise for ten reps.

**Tips:**

Pay attention to maintaining proper alignment throughout the exercise. Keep your back straight, engage your core, and avoid any forward lean.

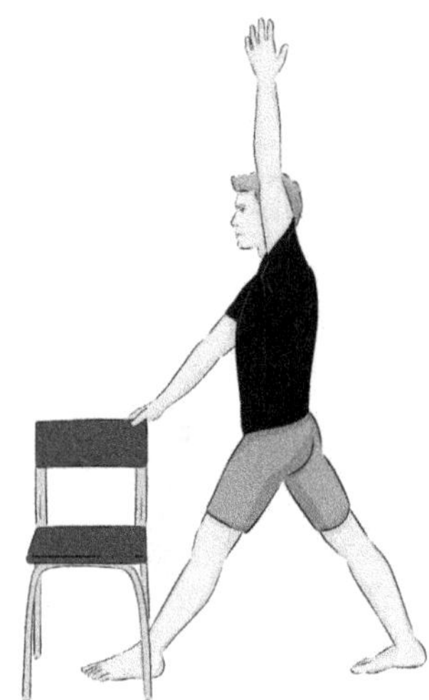

1. Position a sturdy chair in front of you, ensuring it's on a stable surface. Stand with your feet hip-width apart and place your hands on the backrest of the chair for support.

2. Reach your right arm forward and hold onto the backrest of the chair. Keep a soft bend in the right elbow to avoid locking the joint.

3. Inhale deeply as you extend your left arm overhead, reaching toward the right side. Your left hand should be in line with your shoulder, forming a straight line from your left fingertips to your left heel.

4. Exhale as you rotate your upper body to the right, opening up your chest. Allow your gaze to follow the movement, looking up toward your left hand.

5. Keep your hips facing forward, avoiding any rotation. This emphasizes the stretch along the left side of your body, from your fingertips down to your left heel.

6. Hold the extended position for fifteen seconds, feeling a deep stretch along the left side. Do this exercise for five reps.

7. Repeat on the other side.

**Tips:**

Focus on keeping a stable foundation by engaging your core and maintaining a strong connection with the floor through your feet.

# AWARENESS IN MOVEMENT EXERCISES

The following exercises to follow are a bit more intense than those in the previous section. They place more resistance stress on your muscles while also challenging your mobility and proprioception.

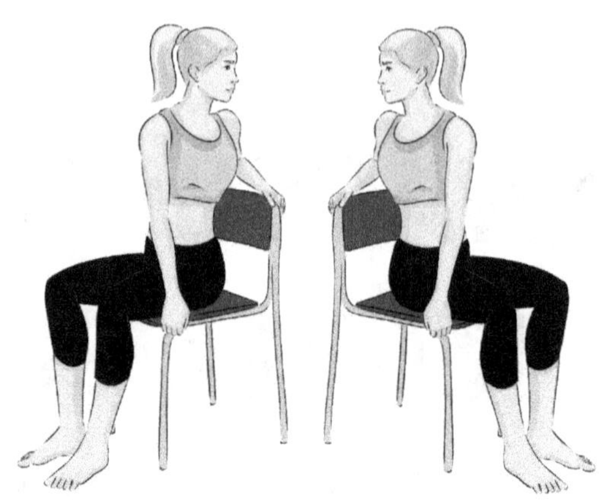

1 Sit down on a chair or on the ground with your back straight and chest up.

2 Place your arm on the backrest of the chair and, as you lengthen your spine, turn backward as far as you comfortably can.

3 Now return to center and turn to the other side. Do twelve reps on each side.

**Tips:**

Don't sacrifice the turn distance for bad form or by twisting and tightening your core or your spine. Instead, gain length by visualizing extending your spine.

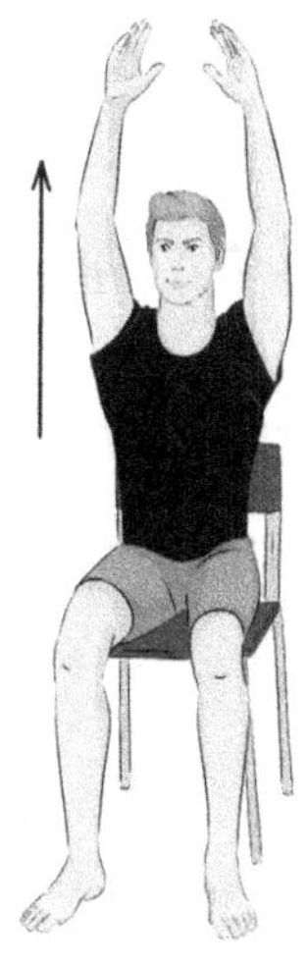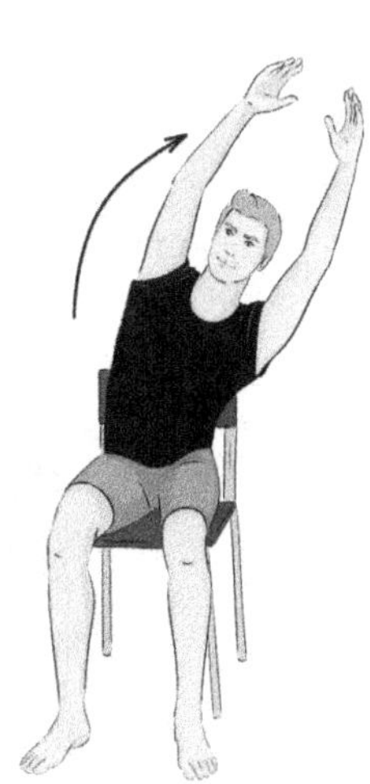

1   Sit up straight on a chair with your feet flat on the floor and your hands raised high up in the air.

2   Take a few breaths and lengthen your spine. As you do, lean to the right with your hands leading.

3   Now return to center and turn to the other side. Perform ten reps on each side.

**Tips:**

Don't sacrifice the leaning distance by tightening muscles. Gain mobility by lengthening your muscles.

# Chair Arm Circles

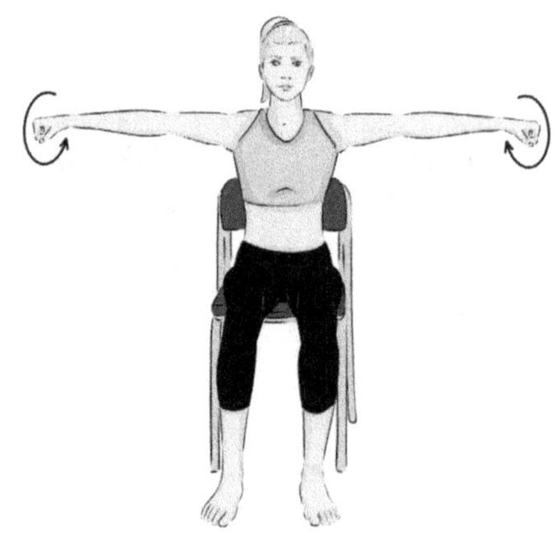

1 Sit up straight on a chair with your feet flat on the floor. Extend your arms straight out to the sides, parallel to the floor.

2 Begin making small circular motions with your arms, like you're drawing circles with your hands.

3 You can use an open-handed palm or your fists.

4 Continue the circular motions for ten seconds. Now, go in the other direction for ten seconds.

5 Do five repetitions of this exercise.

**Tips:**

- Maintain slow and controlled movements to avoid straining your shoulders.

- Gradually increase the size of the circles as you feel comfortable.

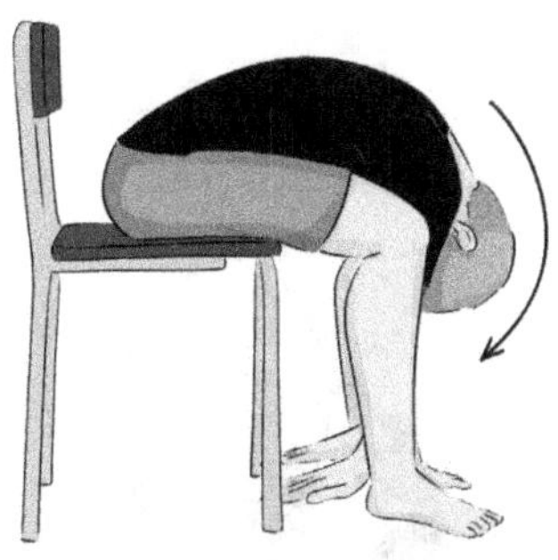

1. Sit upright with your feet flat on the floor. Sit toward the front edge of the chair to allow space for the forward bend.

2. Activate your core by drawing your navel toward your spine. This engagement supports the movement and protects your lower back.

3. Inhale deeply, lengthening your spine and reaching the crown of your head toward the ceiling. Keep your shoulders relaxed and down, away from your ears.

4. As you exhale, hinge at your hips and begin to lean forward from your waist. Lead with your chest, allowing your torso to descend toward your thighs. Keep your back straight throughout the movement.

5. Extend your arms forward, reaching toward the floor or the space between your feet. If reaching the floor is challenging, aim to touch your shins or the sides of your feet.

6. Hold the forward bend for fifteen seconds, feeling a gentle stretch along your spine, hamstrings, and hips. Focus on relaxing into the stretch and breathing deeply.

7. Inhale as you slowly return to an upright seated position, engaging your core to support the ascent.

8. Do five reps of this exercise.

**Tips:**

If you're new to this exercise, start with a smaller range of motion and gradually progress as your flexibility increases. Avoid bouncing or forcing the stretch to prevent injury.

# Chair Tree Pose

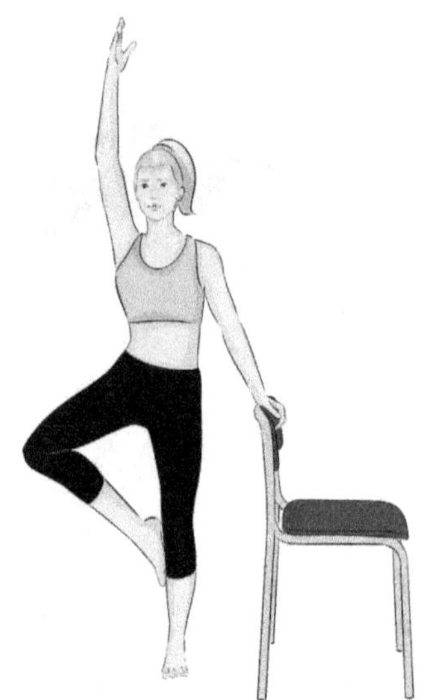

1. Begin by placing a sturdy chair next to you. Stand tall with your feet hip-width apart, arms by your sides, and shoulders relaxed.

2. Transfer your weight onto your left leg while keeping a slight bend in the knee. This is your standing leg for the tree pose.

3. Bend your right knee and bring the sole of your right foot to rest on the inner left thigh or calf. Avoid placing the foot directly on the knee to protect the joint.

4. Hold onto the backrest of the chair with your right hand for support.

5. Bring your left arm overhead so that your hand is directly above your head.

6. Stay in the tree pose for twenty to thirty seconds or longer if comfortable. Focus on your breath and find a focal point to enhance balance.

7. Repeat on the opposite side.

8. Do five reps of this exercise.

**Tips:**

If you're new to the tree pose, start with the foot resting on the calf instead of the inner thigh. As your balance improves, gradually work your way up to the full expression of the pose.

# Chair Goddess Pose

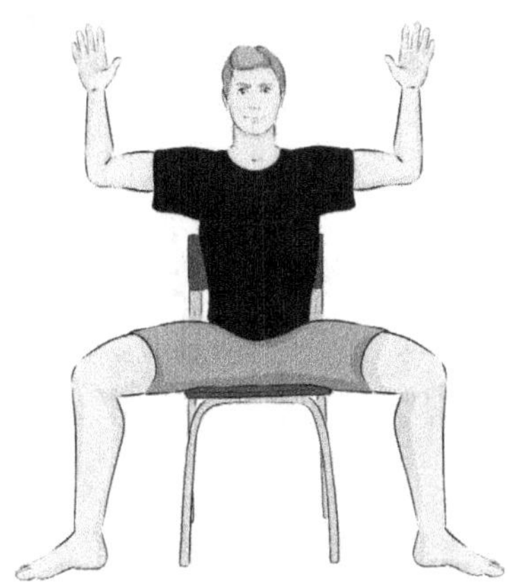

1. Sit on the edge of the chair with your feet shoulder-width apart.

2. Slide your feet outward, opening your knees to the sides. Aim to bring your thighs parallel to the floor, forming a wide "V" shape with your legs.

3. Turn your toes slightly outward to accommodate the opening of the knees. Ensure your feet remain flat on the floor.

4. Bring your arms up to the "hands up" position. Push your shoulder blades down and extend your chest out in this position.

5. Hold the chair goddess pose for twenty seconds.

6. Do five reps of this exercise.

**Tips:**

Pay attention to the alignment of your knees over your ankles. Ensure that your knees track in line with your toes to protect the joints and promote proper engagement of the muscles.

# Chair Goddess Twist

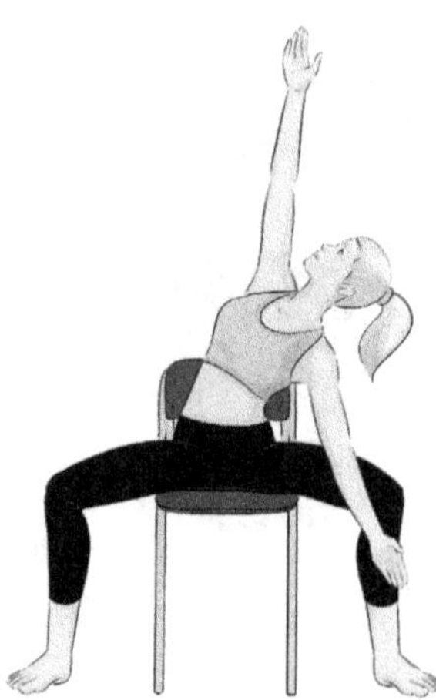

1. Sit on the edge of the chair with your feet shoulder-width apart.

2. Slide your feet outward, opening your knees to the sides. Aim to bring your thighs parallel to the floor, forming a wide "V" shape with your legs.

3. Turn your toes slightly outward to accommodate the opening of the knees. Ensure your feet remain flat on the floor.

4. Bring your arms up to the "hands up" position. Push your shoulder blades down and extend your chest out in this position.

5. Engage your core by drawing your navel toward your spine.

6. Exhale as you begin to twist your upper body to the right, bringing your left hand up and overhead.

7. Turn your head to look up toward your extended hand.

8. Hold this position for fifteen seconds, breathing deeply and maintaining engagement in your core.

9. Inhale as you slowly return to the center, bringing your arms overhead again.

10. Repeat on the other side.

11. Do five reps of this exercise.

**Tips:**

Focus on controlled and deliberate movements during the twist. Avoid jerky motions to protect your spine and maintain balance.

# Reverse Tabletop

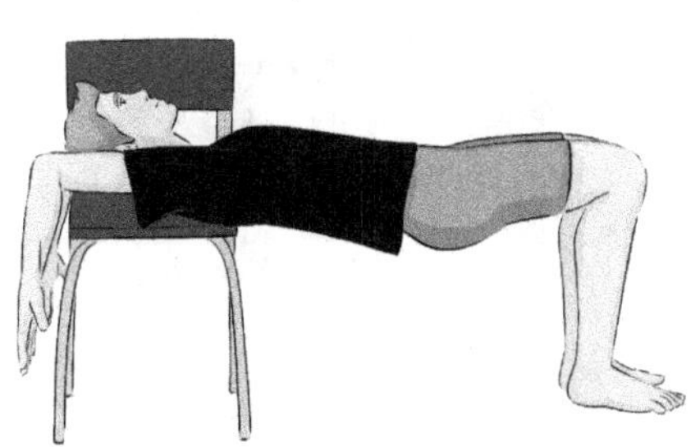

1. Position yourself on the edge of a sturdy chair with your feet flat on the floor. Place your hands on the chair, fingers pointing toward your feet, and ensure they are shoulder-width apart.

2. Bend your knees and place your feet hip-width apart on the floor, keeping your ankles directly below your knees.

3. Press into your hands on the chair and lift your hips toward the ceiling, creating a reverse tabletop position. Your torso and thighs should form a straight line parallel to the floor.

4. Allow your head to gently drop back, opening your chest by squeezing your shoulder blades together. Ensure your neck is comfortable and there's no strain.

5. Extend your hands overhead and bend your elbows so that they are alongside your ears.

6. Tighten your core muscles to maintain a straight line from your shoulders to your knees. Be mindful of avoiding excessive arching in the lower back.

7. Hold the extended position for fifteen seconds.

8. Repeat on the other side.

9. Do five reps of this exercise.

**Tips:**

Ensure the chair is stable and positioned on a nonslip surface.

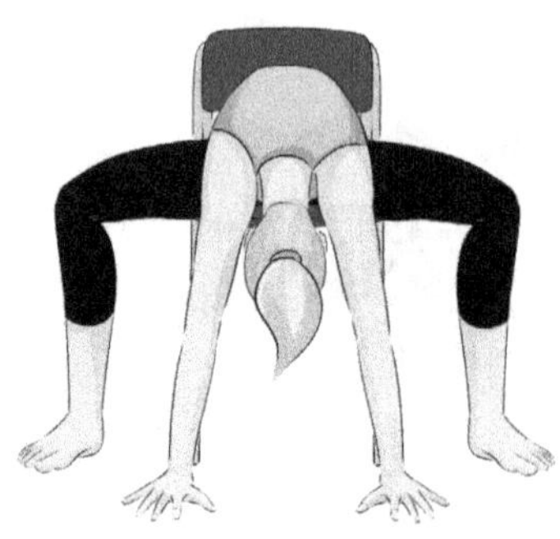

1. Sit on the edge of a sturdy chair with your knees out wide and toes pointed outward.

2. Inhale deeply as you lengthen your spine, raising your arms overhead. Keep your shoulders relaxed and away from your ears.

3. As you exhale, hinge at your hips and begin to fold forward from your waist. Maintain a straight back as you lead with your chest. Reach your hands toward the floor.

4. Allow your neck and shoulders to relax. Your head can hang naturally, or you can gaze forward, depending on your comfort level.

5. Hold the Forward Fold: Hold the seated wide-legged forward fold for twenty seconds, breathing deeply and allowing your body to release tension.

6. Inhale as you slowly rise back to an upright seated position, keeping your back straight.

7. Do five reps of this exercise.

**Tips:**

Depending on the chair's height, you may need to place a cushion on the chair or adjust your positioning to ensure a comfortable and effective stretch.

# Seated Warrior III Pose

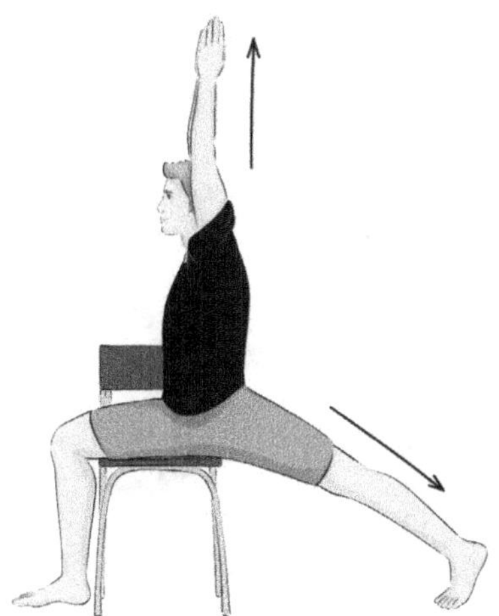

1. Begin by sitting side-on in a sturdy chair with your feet flat on the floor and your left foot in front. Sit tall, engaging your core and keeping your spine straight.

2. Shift your weight onto your left foot, firmly planting it into the ground. Extend your right leg behind you, planting the balls of your feet on the floor.

3. Reach your hands overhead to touch your fingertips above your head. Stretch through your upper back as you hold the pose. Tighten your core muscles to maintain balance and stability. Focus on pulling your navel toward your spine.

4. Hold the seated Warrior III pose for fifteen to thirty seconds or longer if comfortable. Keep breathing steadily and maintain a strong, controlled posture.

5. Repeat on the other side.

6. Do five reps of this exercise.

**Tips:**

Start with a shorter duration and gradually increase the time spent in the pose as your strength and balance improve. Consistency is key to progress.

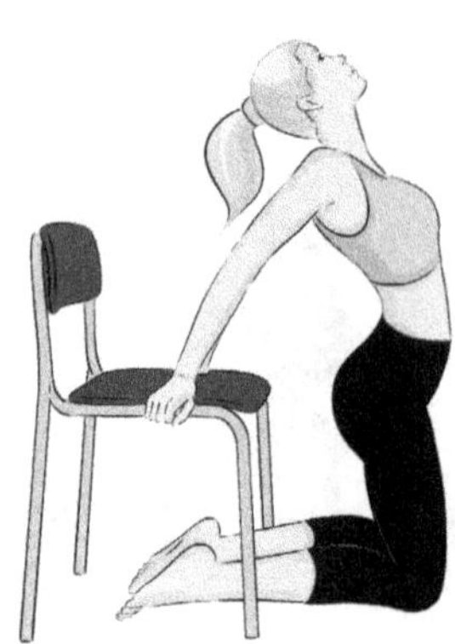

1  Kneel on the floor with your knees hip-width apart. Place a sturdy chair behind you, ensuring it won't slide. The chair should be close enough for your hands to comfortably rest on it without straining your shoulders.

2  Kneel with your shins and the tops of your feet pressing into the floor. Ensure your knees are directly below your hips.

3  Reach your hands back and place them on the chair, fingers pointing downward. Keep your hands shoulder-width apart and your fingers spread for a stable grip.

4  Inhale deeply, and as you exhale, begin to lean backward. Lift your chest toward the ceiling, opening the front of your body.

5  Hold the Chair Camel Pose for thirty seconds, breathing steadily. Focus on lengthening your spine and opening your chest.

6  Inhale as you gently return to an upright kneeling position.

7  Do five reps of this exercise.

**Tips:**

Choose a chair that allows your hands to comfortably rest on it without causing strain on your shoulders. The height of the chair can impact the intensity of the stretch, so adjust as needed.

# GENTLE MOMENTUM EXERCISES

The exercises in this section focus on specific muscles through their full range of motion. You will use gentle momentum to extend your flexibility and strength while also increasing your heart rate.

# Cross Leg Side Bend

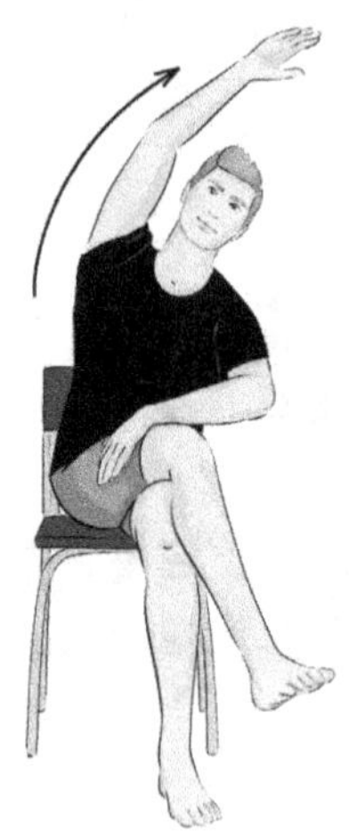

1 Sit with your back straight and your feet flat on the floor, hip-width apart.

2 Bring your right ankle to rest on top of your left knee. If this is uncomfortable, simply cross your legs at the ankles.

3 Inhale as you lengthen your spine, sitting up tall. Imagine your head reaching towards the ceiling.

4 Place your right hand on your left knee and raise your left arm over.

5 Gently stretch your torso to the right by bringing your right arm over your head. Feel the stretch along the right side of your torso.

6 Hold the stretch for fifteen seconds, breathing deeply and maintaining a comfortable level of tension.

7 Repeat on the other side.

8 Do five reps on this exercise.

**Tips:**

Keep your shoulders relaxed and avoid collapsing into the stretch.

# Leg and Arm Lift

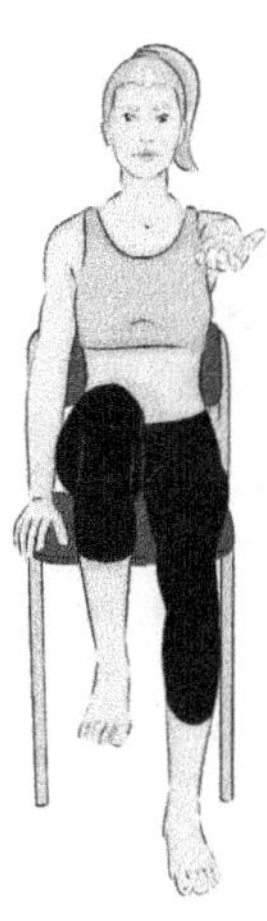

1. Sit with your back straight and your feet flat on the floor, hip-width apart. Relax your shoulders and place your hands on your knees.

2. Inhale as you lift your right arm forward and up to shoulder height. Keep your palm facing upward.

3. Simultaneously lift your left foot off the ground by about twelve inches.

4. Hold the raised arm and leg position for five seconds, maintaining your balance. Focus on a point in front of you to help with stability.

5. Repeat with the opposite arm and leg.

6. Do five reps on this exercise.

**Tips:**

Focus on controlled and deliberate movements rather than speed. This exercise is about maintaining balance and control.

# Chair Boat Pose

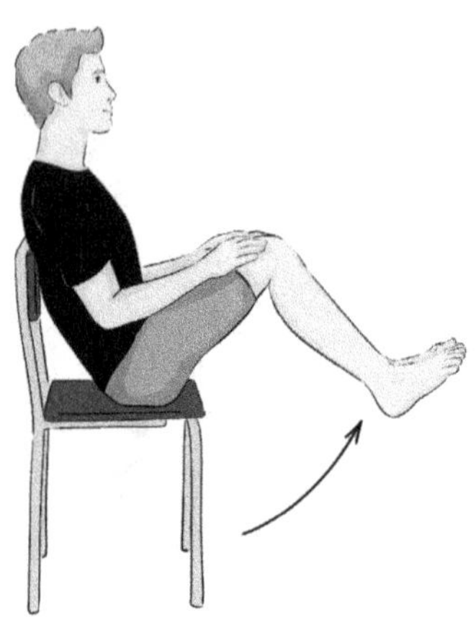

1  Sit with your back straight and your feet flat on the floor, hip-width apart. Now slide forward to the edge of the chair.

2  Inhale as you lift your feet off the ground, bringing your shins parallel to the floor. Your knees should be bent at a 90-degree angle.

3  Place your hands on your knees.

4  Shift your weight onto your sit bones, finding balance on the edge of the chair. Keep your back straight and your chest lifted.

5  Hold the Chair Boat Pose for fifteen seconds, focusing on your breath and maintaining a stable position.

6  Do five reps on this exercise.

**Tips:**

To maximize the benefits of this pose, consciously engage your core muscles. Imagine pulling your navel toward your spine to activate the deep abdominal muscles. This not only strengthens your core but also helps with balance.

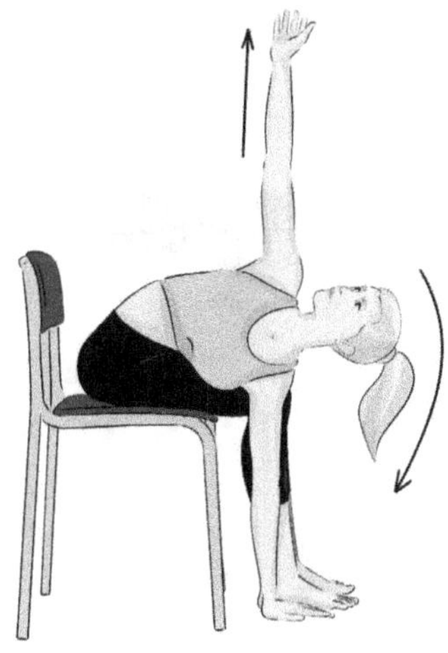

1. Sit with your back straight and your feet flat on the floor hip-width apart.

2. Inhale deeply as you lengthen your spine, sitting up tall. Imagine your head reaching toward the ceiling.

3. Exhale as you twist your torso to the right and down, bringing your left hand down to the floor. Simultaneously, lift your right hand toward the ceiling.

4. Hold the twist for a count of five, feeling the stretch along the spine. Keep your shoulders relaxed and your neck in line with your spine as you look up toward your extended hand.

5. Inhale as you return to the center, bringing your spine back to a neutral position.

6. Repeat on the other side.

7. Do five reps on this exercise.

**Tips:**

Focus on gentle and controlled movements to avoid strain. Ensure that your spine is aligned and the twist comes from your waist, not your shoulders. This helps target the muscles along the spine and encourages a safe stretch.

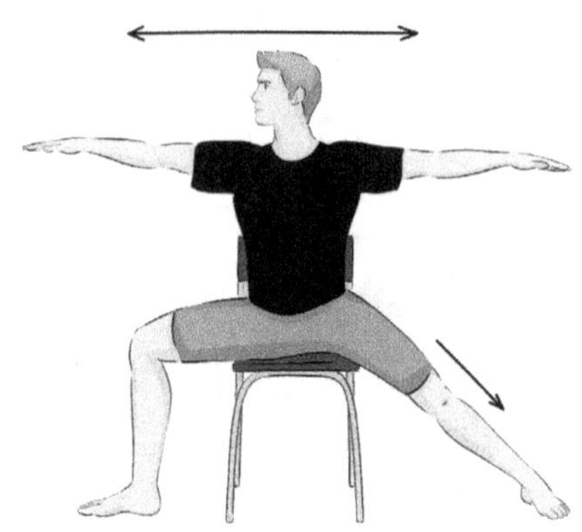

1  Begin by sitting side-on a sturdy chair with your feet flat on the floor and your left foot in front. Sit tall, engaging your core and keeping your spine straight.

2  Shift your weight onto your left foot, firmly planting it into the ground. Extend your right leg behind you, planting the balls of your feet on the floor.

3  Reach your arms out directly in line with your shoulders. Stretch through your upper back as you hold the pose. Tighten your core muscles to maintain balance and stability. Focus on pulling your navel toward your spine.

4  Hold the seated Warrior II pose for fifteen seconds or longer if comfortable. Keep breathing steadily and maintain a strong, controlled posture.

5  Repeat on the other side.

6  Do five reps on this exercise.

**Tips:**

Start with a shorter duration and gradually increase the time spent in the pose as your strength and balance improve. Consistency is key to progress.

# Chair Reverse Warrior

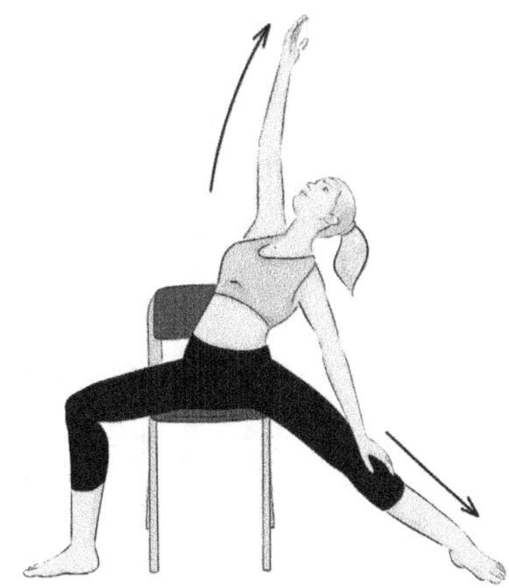

1 Start in a sitting position with your feet three to four feet apart with the chair in the middle as a stabilizer.

2 Turn your left foot out while your right foot straightens out to the side. Extend your arms out to the sides.

3 Bend your left knee to a 90-degree angle while keeping your right leg straight. Keep your torso facing forward and gaze over your left hand.

4 Hold the warrior pose here for five seconds. Now, move your right hand upward and to the left as far as you comfortably can.

5 Hold for five seconds.

6 Now repeat this for the other side (right foot 90-degree angle, left foot straight).

7 Do this exercise for five reps.

**Tips:**

As you get stronger, you can do this without the chair.

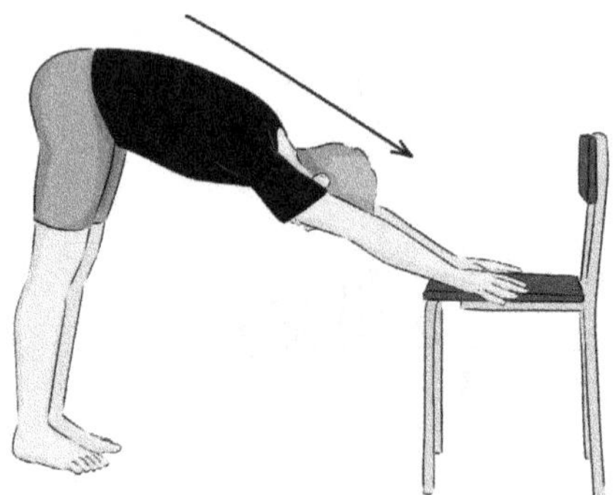

1. Stand facing your chair, about three feet away from it, with your feet hip-width apart, ensuring a comfortable and stable stance.

2. Hinge at your hips, reaching forward with your hands to grasp the sides of the chair. Your arms should be extended, and your spine should be straight.

3. Take a few steps back to create a diagonal line from your hands to your hips. Your body should form an inverted "V" shape. Ensure your feet are parallel to each other and your heels are pressing down into the floor. Your toes can be slightly turned inward.

4. Allow your head to hang naturally between your arms. Keep your neck relaxed, and let your gaze fall between your feet or toward your knees.

5. Hold the pose for fifteen seconds.

6. Do this exercise for five reps.

**Tips:**

Focus on lengthening your spine, reaching your hips toward the ceiling.

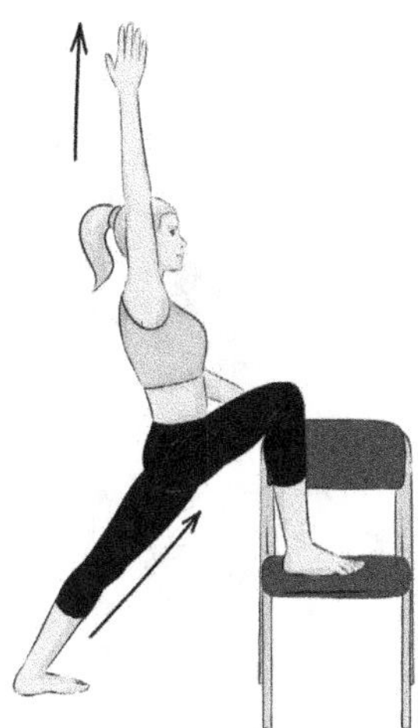

1. Stand side on to a chair, placing your right foot on the chair. Keep your left foot flat on the floor, ensuring it's in line with your hip.

2. Inhale deeply as you lift your right arm overhead, reaching towards the ceiling. Place your left hand on the back of the chair for support.

3. Hold the high lunge position for fifteen seconds, maintaining a strong and stable position. Keep your gaze forward and your chest open.

4. Repeat on the other side.

5. Do this exercise for five reps.

**Tips:**

Concentrate on maintaining stability through the grounded foot and engaged core. This not only enhances the effectiveness of the stretch but also helps improve balance over time.

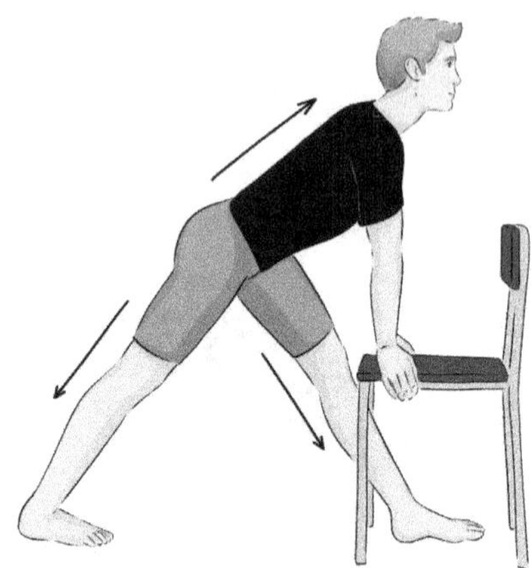

1  Stand in front of a chair with your hands resting on the seat. Stagger your legs so that your right foot is behind and your left foot is between the chair legs. Your feet should be as wide as comfortably possible with your torso at a 45-degree angle.

2  Push into the chair as you extend your spine and look toward the ceiling.

3  Hold the side stretch pose for fifteen seconds, feeling the stretch through your hamstrings and back.

4  Repeat on the other side.

5  Do this exercise for five reps.

**Tips:**

Do not round your back in this movement.

# Seated Extended Side Angle Pose

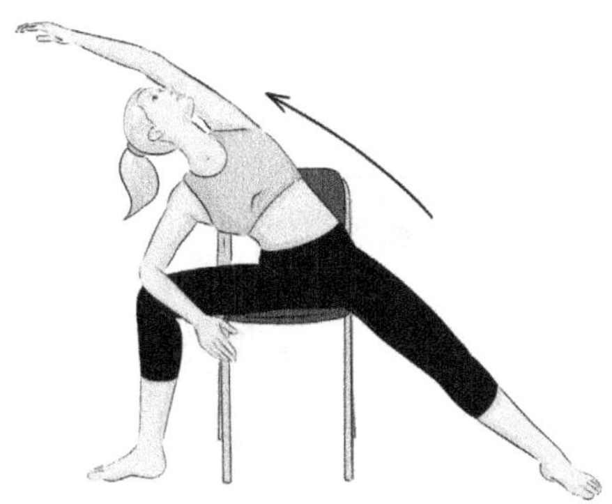

1 Sit with your back straight and your feet flat on the floor, hip-width apart. Slide forward to the edge of the chair.

2 Extend your right leg out to the side, keeping it straight. Your toes should be pointing forward or slightly angled upwards.

3 Keep your left foot firmly planted on the floor, ensuring it's in line with your hip.

4 Inhale deeply as you raise your right arm overhead, reaching towards the ceiling. Rest your right forearm on your right thigh. Your right side should feel a stretch from your fingertips down to your hip.

5 Hold the seated extended side angle pose for fifteen seconds.

6 Repeat on the other side.

7 Do this exercise for five reps.

# Seated Revolved Head-to-Knee Pose

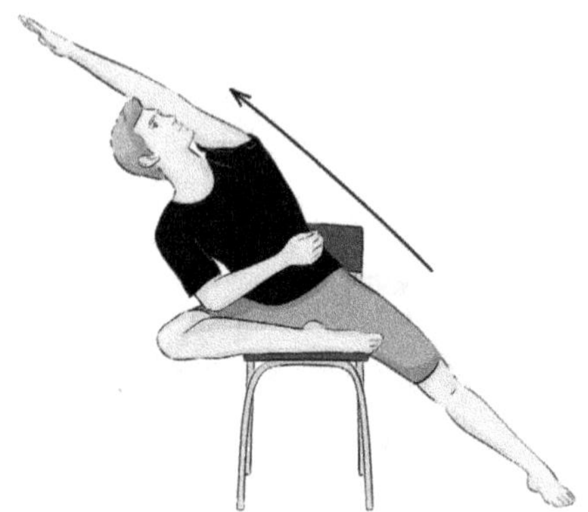

1  Sit with your back straight and your feet flat on the floor, hip-width apart.

2  Scoot forward until you are sitting on the edge of the chair, allowing space behind you.

3  Extend your right leg straight in front.

4  Extend your right leg straight out to the side, keeping it on the floor. Flex your foot to engage the muscles in your right leg.

5  Bend your left knee, bringing the sole of your left foot to the inside of your right thigh so that the lower leg is resting on the chair.

6  Inhale deeply as you raise your right arm overhead, reaching towards the ceiling. Keep your palm facing inward.

7  Exhale and twist towards the right.

8  Hold the pose for fifteen seconds.

9  Repeat on the other side.

**Tips:**

Engage your core throughout the pose to provide stability and support for your lower back. This helps maintain balance and a controlled twist.

# Gate Pose

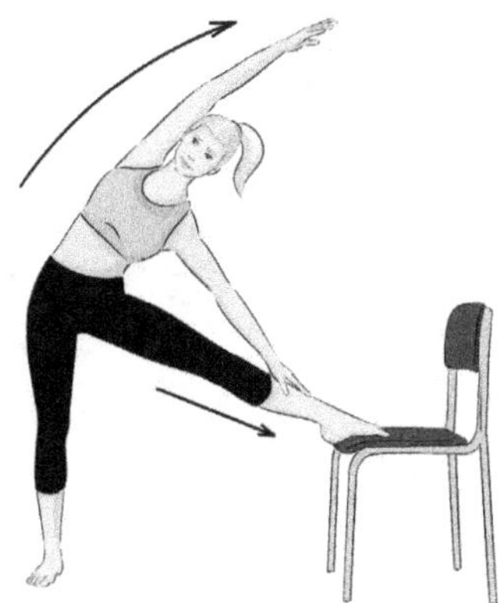

1. Stand side-on to a chair with your feet together and your back straight.

2. Place your closest foot on the chair, resting all of your sole on the seat, with the leg straight.

3. Inhale deeply as you extend your outside arm overhead, reaching towards the ceiling. Bring the inside arm down your leg as far as is comfortable.

4. Hold the pose for fifteen seconds, maintaining a steady breath and feeling the stretch along the left side.

5. Repeat on the other side.

6. Do five reps on this exercise.

**Tips:**

The chair provides stability, so use it as a support throughout the pose. This allows you to focus on the stretch and balance without compromising your stability.

# Seated Crescent High Lunge Twist

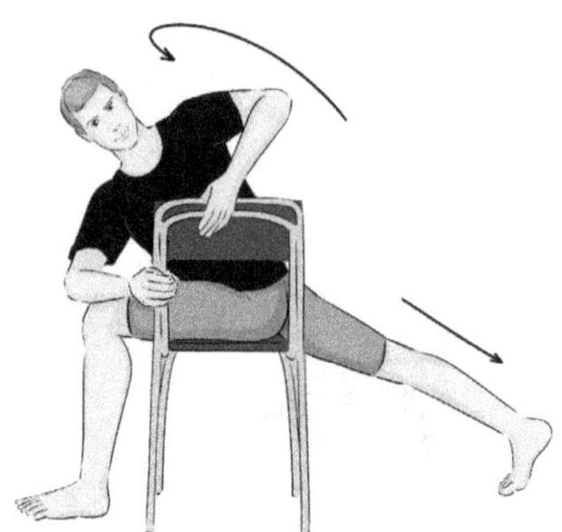

1. Sit with your back straight and your feet flat on the floor hip-width apart.

2. Reach both hands toward the backrest of the chair, holding onto it for support. Ensure your grip is firm and your arms are straight.

3. Inhale as you extend your right leg straight to the side. Point your toes and engage the muscles in your right leg.

4. Keep your left foot flat on the floor, flexing it to create a stable base.

5. Inhale and lengthen your spine.

6. Inhale deeply as you lengthen your spine, sitting up tall.

7. Exhale as you twist your torso to the left, using the chair for support. Allow your chest to open, and bring your right elbow toward the back of the chair.

8. Turn your head to the left, gazing over your left shoulder. Feel the stretch along the spine and the outer hip of your extended right leg.

9. Hold the pose for fifteen seconds, maintaining a strong and stable position.

10. Repeat on the other side.

11. Do five reps on this exercise.

**Tips:**

Throughout the entire exercise, engage your core muscles to provide stability and support for your lower back. This not only enhances the effectiveness of the twist but also helps with balance.

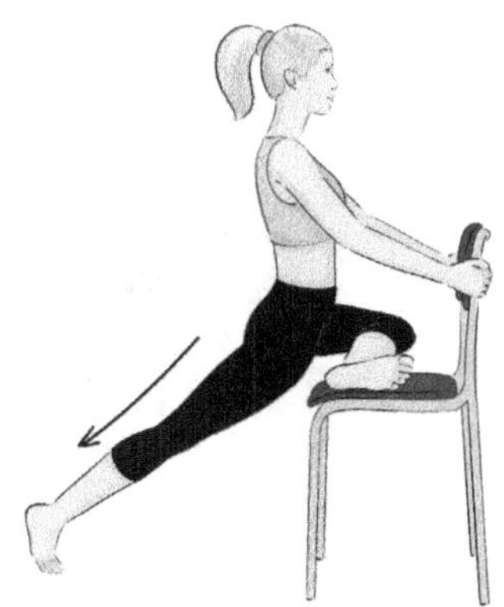

1  Stand in front of a chair, facing it. Bend your left leg to place the lower leg on the chair seat, side on.

2  Reach forward to grab the chair's back edges with both hands.

3  Extend your right leg back behind you as far as you comfortably can, resting on the toes.

4  Pull on the chair back as you lengthen your spine and look toward the ceiling.

5  Hold this pose for fifteen seconds.

6  Do five reps on this exercise.

**Tips:**

Focus on engaging your core muscles throughout the pose. This not only provides stability but also enhances the stretch along the sides of your body.

# Seated Reverse Warrior Pose

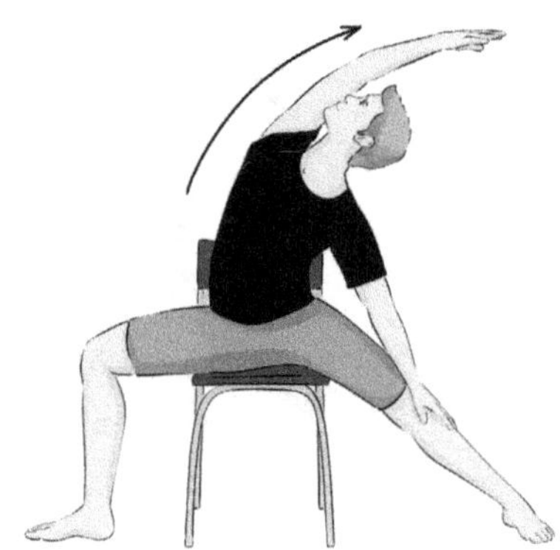

1. Start in a sitting position with your feet three to four feet apart, with the chair in the middle as a stabilizer.

2. Turn your left foot out while your right foot straightens outward to the side.

3. Bend your left knee to a 90-degree angle while keeping your right leg straight. Keep your torso facing forward and gaze over your left hand.

4. Extend your left arm overhead as you tilt your torso to the right, and bring the right arm down your leg as far as you comfortably can.

5. Hold the warrior pose for five seconds.

6. Repeat on the other side.

7. Do this exercise for five reps.

**Tips:**

As you get stronger, you can do this without the chair.

# Mountain Climber

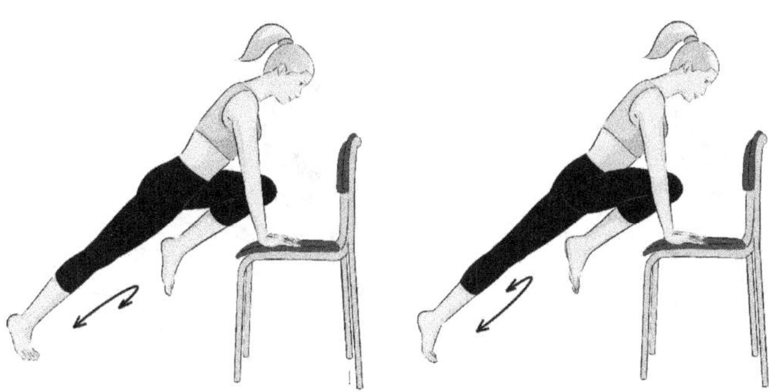

1. Position yourself facing a chair and place your hands on the seat shoulder-width apart.

2. Step back to create a plank position, with your body forming a straight line from head to heels. Keep your wrists directly under your shoulders and your feet hip-width apart.

3. Lean into the chair for added support, distributing your weight evenly between your hands.

4. Lift your right knee toward your chest, engaging your core muscles. Alternate legs in a dynamic and controlled manner, simulating a running motion. Focus on bringing your knees as close to your chest as comfortably possible.

5. Perform the mountain climber at a pace that challenges you but allows for proper form. Maintain a smooth, controlled rhythm to enhance the effectiveness of the exercise.

6. Perform fifteen repetitions on each leg.

**Tips:**

Focus on engaging your abdominal muscles throughout the exercise. Tighten your core as you perform the mountain climber to enhance stability and target the muscles in your abdomen.

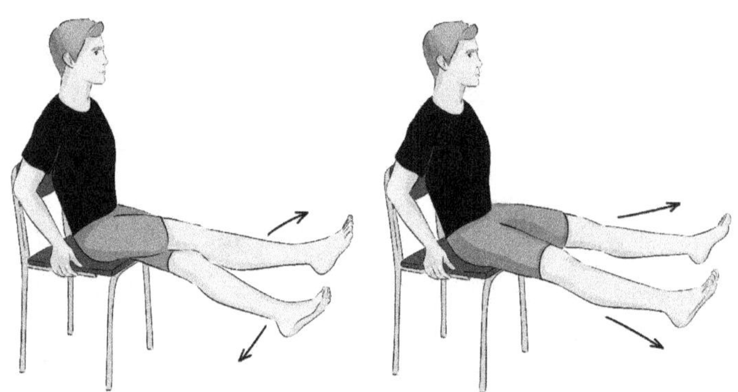

1 Sit on a chair with your back straight and your legs extended in front of you, hip-width apart. Grasp the sides of the chair for support.

2 Lift both feet slightly off the ground and begin to shuffle them across each other in scissor fashion. Continue this side-to-side shuffling motion.

3 Perform the shuffling movement at a controlled and deliberate pace. Focus on maintaining balance and control throughout the exercise, avoiding any sudden or jerky movements.

4 Do fifteen repetitions of this exercise.

**Tips:**

As you shuffle your feet, engage your core muscles to maintain stability. This adds an extra element to the exercise, promoting abdominal strength and stability.

# Chair Rotation Step and Reach

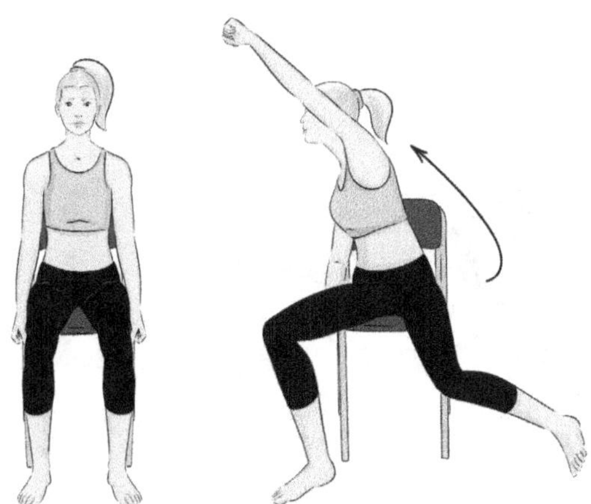

1  Sit comfortably on a chair with your feet flat on the floor hip-width apart. Ensure proper posture with your spine straight and your shoulders relaxed.

2  Begin with your hands resting on the sides of the chair seat. Engage your core by drawing your navel toward your spine.

3  Inhale deeply, and as you exhale, lift your right foot slightly off the floor. Simultaneously, rotate your torso to the left, reaching across and up with your right arm. Your left hand can slide along your left thigh for support.

4  Extend your right arm diagonally across your body and upward, reaching toward the left side. Feel a gentle rotation through your torso.

5  Hold the extended reach for a moment, breathing deeply. Feel the stretch along your side, through the arm, and across the torso.

6  Repeat on the other side.

7  Do ten reps on this exercise.

**Tips:**

Focus on the smoothness and control of the movement. Avoid jerky motions and allow the stretch to be gradual.

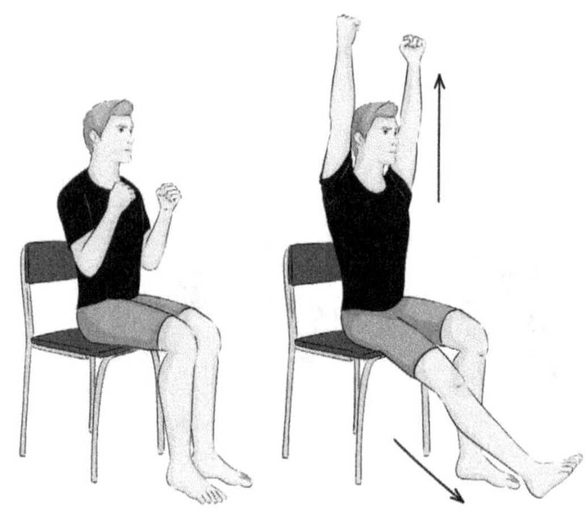

1 Sit comfortably on a chair with your back straight and feet flat on the floor, hip-width apart. Ensure a stable base and relaxed shoulders.

2 Bring your hands to your heart center, palms pressed together. Engage your core muscles by drawing your navel toward your spine.

3 Inhale deeply, and as you exhale, step your right foot forward, extending it in front of you. Maintain stability by keeping your weight centered over your hips.

4 Simultaneously, extend both arms overhead in a pressing motion.

Keep your palms facing each other, and fully extend your arms without locking the elbows.

5 Lower and repeat.

6 Do fifteen reps of this exercise.

**Tips:**

Hold the extended position for a moment, feeling the stretch through the arms and the engagement of the leg muscles. Maintain steady breathing throughout the movement.

# UNWINDING RELAXATION EXERCISES

The cool-down exercises in this section are designed to gently return your body to its relaxed, pre-exercise state. They also promote a calm, meditative mental state.

# Elbow Reach

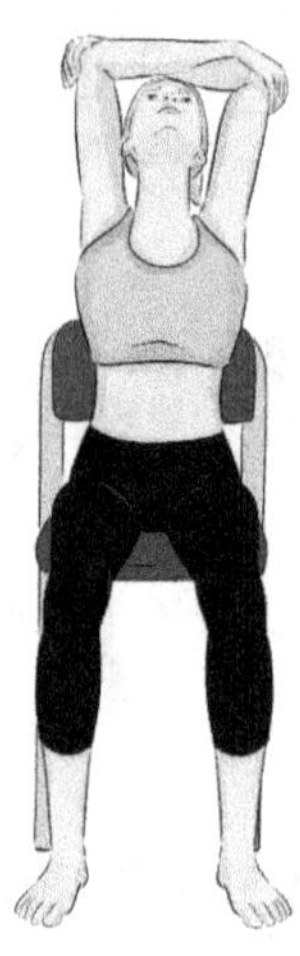

1. Sit comfortably on a chair with your feet flat on the floor, hip-width apart. Ensure that your back is straight and your shoulders are relaxed.

2. Extend your arms overhead, then bend your elbows so that your forearms are parallel to the floor. Place your hands over the opposite elbow.

3. Expand your chest and reach up into the stretch.

4. Hold the pose for thirty seconds, feeling a comfortable stretch.

**Tips:**

Pay attention to your breath and initiate the stretch on the exhale. Exhaling while stretching upward helps activate your core muscles and allows for a deeper stretch.

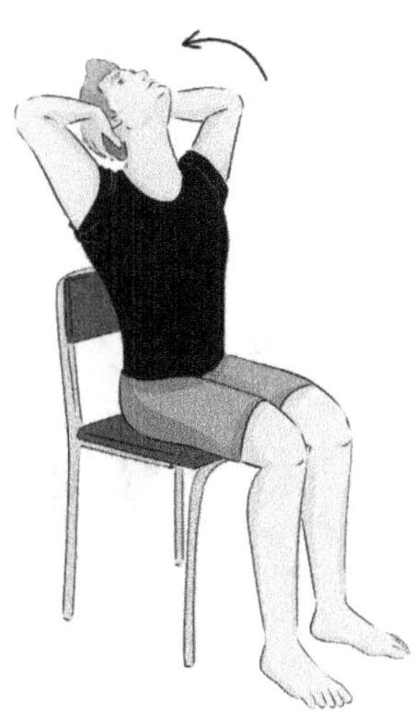

1 Begin by sitting side-on a sturdy chair with your feet flat on the floor and your left foot in front. Sit tall, engaging your core and keeping your spine straight.

2 Place your hands by your ears.

3 Inhale deeply as you lengthen your spine. As you exhale, gently arch your upper back, allowing your head to lean back and be supported by the top of the chair's backrest.

4 Hold this pose for thirty seconds.

5 Do this exercise five times.

**Tips:**

Focus on the quality of the stretch rather than the depth of the arch. It's important to maintain a comfortable and pain-free range of motion. If you experience any discomfort or strain, reduce the intensity of the arch.

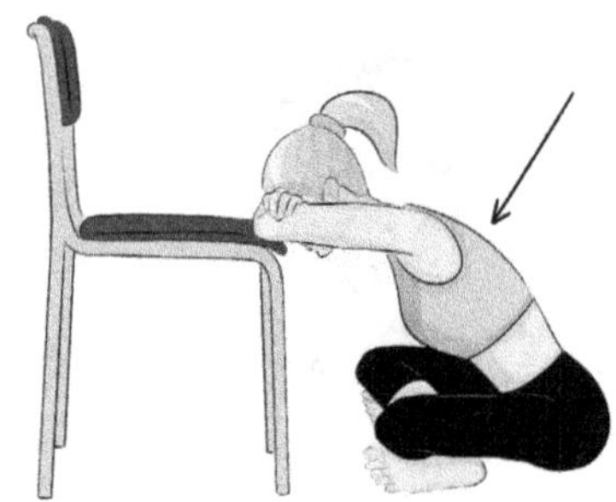

1. Sit on the floor facing a chair with your legs crossed.

2. Gently lower your upper body to rest on the chair seat. Your arms and head should comfortably rest on the chair, allowing for a supported and relaxed position.

3. Close your eyes and focus on your breath. Inhale deeply through your nose, allowing your belly to rise, and exhale slowly through your mouth.

Embrace the stillness and take this moment for relaxation.

4. Remain in this seated rest position for five minutes, allowing your body to relax and release tension.

**Tips:**

Use a cushion under your hips if you find the floor uncomfortable.

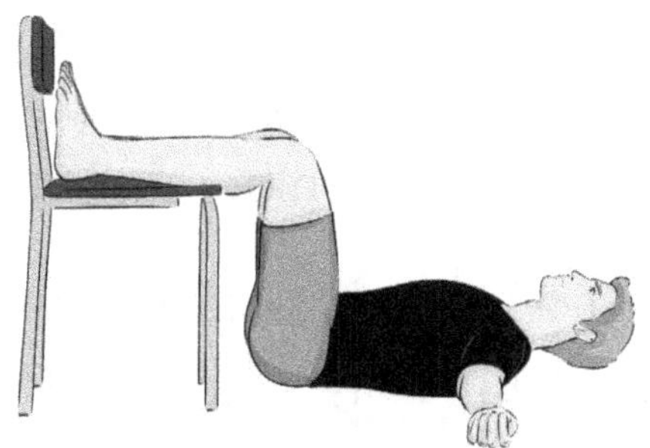

1. Sit on the ground in front of a chair facing it. Your knees should be bent, your feet flat on the floor, and your arms resting by your sides.

2. Gently lower yourself onto your back, keeping your knees bent. Use your hands to support your descent.

3. Lift your legs and place them on the seat of the chair. Your calves and heels should be supported, creating a right angle with your knees.

4. Scoot your hips close to the chair to ensure your legs are well supported. Your lower back should be resting comfortably on the ground.

5. Relax your arms.

6. Allow your arms to rest out to the sides, palms facing up. This position promotes an open chest and relaxation.

7. Close your eyes to enhance the relaxation response. Focus on your breath and let go of any tension.

8. Hold the pose for five minutes, allowing your body to unwind and your muscles to release tension.

**Tips:**

Utilize deep, diaphragmatic breathing to enhance relaxation. Inhale slowly through your nose, allowing your abdomen to rise, and exhale fully through your mouth or nose. Deep breathing promotes relaxation, reduces stress, and helps release tension in the lower back and legs.

# Next Steps

As we conclude our journey through chair yoga exercises for weight loss, I hope you've discovered the incredible transformative power of these gentle yet effective movements. Congratulations on committing to this path of wellness!

This guide has provided you with a structured and motivating framework to incorporate chair yoga into your daily routine. The positive changes you've experienced so far are only the beginning.

After a while, regular chair yoga exercises will make you feel more flexible, stronger, toned, and more vibrant in every way. You've laid the foundation for a healthier and more active lifestyle, and the benefits will continue to unfold with each passing day.

As you progress, remember that consistency is key. After about eight weeks, this will become a habit for the rest of your life. Your commitment to these exercises has set the stage for lasting well-being, and I encourage you to stay dedicated to your health and fitness journey.

Thank you for joining me on this chair yoga adventure. Your dedication to self-care is truly commendable. May your journey toward a healthier, happier you continue to flourish. Remember, the benefits of these exercises extend far beyond physical fitness—they are a gift to your mind, body, and spirit.

I know that some of you will want to continue onto more advanced exercises, so before we say goodbye, let me direct you to our exclusive pelvic floor Kegels exercise guide at wallpilates.org as taught by Tim Sawyer, a leading physical therapist who worked with Dr. Anderson and Dr. Wise at the Stanford University Medical Center[*].  When you enter your email to download this free bonus, you'll

---

[*]    Authors of *A Headache in the Pelvis: A New Understanding and Treatment for Chronic Pelvic Pain Syndromes.*

also be notified of new Pilates books and workout routines we'll release in the future.

You can also scan the following QR code to receive your free bonus:

Wishing you continued success on your wellness journey.

Namaste.

# Thank You

My name is Luna, and it has been my pleasure to serve you. You could have picked from dozens of other books, but you took a chance and chose this one. So, thank you for investing in yourself and making it to the end!

Before we say goodbye, one question: If you enjoyed this book, would you consider leaving a review? A review is the easiest and best way to support the work of independent authors like me. Your feedback will help us continue writing the types of books that will help you and others in the journey to good health.

**You can leave a review in fifteen seconds (and get your free bonus):**

https://www.wallpilates.org/

To your happiness and health—Luna Light

# BOOK 2

# CHAIR YOGA
## FOR SENIORS

*28-Day Challenge to Lose Weight, Improve Posture, Balance, Mobility, & Strength in 10 Minutes a Day*

# Contents

# The **Problem** of Aging

**_"Old age is a shipwreck."_**
— _Charles de Gaulle_

After the age of fifty, the human body experiences many changes that make it easier to gain weight, lose muscle, and have poorer posture.

It starts with a decline in testosterone and growth hormones. On average, between ages 30 and 70, testosterone declines by 1–2 percent a year. One to two percent might not sound like much, but that's a 20 percent decline by age 50 and a 40 percent decline by age 70![*] With lower testosterone, muscle mass tends to decrease, and fat mass tends to increase. Because the muscles control movements in our joints, bone health issues (osteoporosis) start occurring. Less growth hormones also mean muscle repair and recovery are slower, so workouts don't feel as fun as they used to during and afterward.

In America, our mobility and flexibility are further limited by a prolonged sedentary lifestyle and an increase in reliance on technology. Because our city infrastructure requires cars to get around, we sit around more in them instead of walking, we watch more and more TV, stare at our phones with Internet access, and over the years... our mobility starts to decline, slowly at first and faster as time accumulates.

Yet, for every case of limited mobility and dwindling health, there are 50, 60, 70, and 80-year-olds with vibrant energy who feel freedom in their movements.

My dad is 72. He plays golf on Mondays, hangs out with friends on Tuesdays, and plays the saxophone with his elder group on Wednesdays. Every morning and

---

[*]     B. R. Zirkin and J. L. Tenover. "Aging and declining testosterone past, present, and hopes for the future." _Journal of Andrology._ (2012). 1111–1118. https://www.ncbi.nlm.nih.gov/pmc/articles/PMC4077344/

evening, he takes a brisk walk around his house. Mom follows him around when she feels like it. Otherwise, she's tending to her garden—digging, planting, and selling the vegetables she grows mostly for recreation.

In addition to my parents, many senior students of mine who practice yoga, Pilates, and somatic movements (low-risk, low-impact forms of exercise) with gentle movement techniques all retain their physical and mental functions despite aging bodies.

That's why if you want to feel lighter, healthier, and have more freedom with your body, you're in luck! This book will help you discover a holistic solution to rebuilding your body using chair yoga, no matter how old you are.

# **The** Solution

> *"You are never too old to set another goal or to dream a new dream."*
> *— C. S. Lewis*

Chair yoga is the reason you bought this book.

But chair yoga itself is NOT the answer. Before you start looking for the refund page on Amazon, let me explain: Chair yoga is just a tool for us to get to the real solution.

What is the real solution to weight loss, limited mobility, and bad posture as we age?

In my humble opinion, it's a holistic approach of proper alignment, movement, and exercise that gives freedom to your body's movements. And in order to start this process, we're going to focus on the chair.

Why the chair? Because the chair helps us do three things really well:

First, it provides **instant feedback.** We can feel how strong we're pushing against an object, and we can add resistance training against it.

Second, the chair gives us **stability;** it's an object to stand, move, and exercise our muscles around even if we have limited mobility, whether sitting down or using it as a stabilizer while standing.

Third, the chair can help us become **aware of our spinal alignment and posture.** I'll show you how to do this using the principles of the Alexander technique in the first group of exercises.

# "Why Should I Listen to You, Luna?"

*"The only disability in life is a bad attitude."*
— Scott Hamilton, Olympic figure skater and cancer survivor

You might be wondering who I am and why you should listen to me.

Hi, I'm Luna. I'm a Pilates and yoga teacher who recovered from a car accident using the exercises I'm about to teach you.

Five years ago, I was in an accident that left me in so much pain that I could not walk and was restricted to a small bedroom at a friend's house. Necessity forced me to discover new ways of exercising and getting my life back.

Over the next year, I started learning about ways to exercise and strengthen my body by using low-impact but highly effective training. I learned about Pilates, yoga, and somatic movements.

It took a long time, but I recovered from my chronic pain using a combination of these soothing movements. As I continued to strengthen my body, I was surprised to find that the pain was gone, and I continued to get stronger and more flexible and had better posture than I had before the accident!

Chair yoga is simple and easy, and if you're mobility-restricted offers a gentle way to strengthen your body. You can do it in the comfort of your home.

## Trigger Point Check

One thing you should look into if you're not seeing improvement is to check for trigger points where you sense muscle pain or weakness. If you have active trigger points, exercising the muscle does not solve the problem. In this case, I highly recommend The Trigger Point Therapy Workbook by the late Clair Davies.

If you have trigger points, our goal is to **1)** clear any trigger points in your muscles and then **2)** use low-risk, low-impact but efficient exercise movements to regain strength. By doing it in this order, you will become tension-free and stronger.

The movements in this book only take fifteen to twenty minutes a day. And all it takes is two weeks for this to become a feel-good habit.


Love,

*Luna Light*

**I wanted to take a moment to remind you that your book comes with a free bonus e-book: *Ultimate Kegels Guide.***

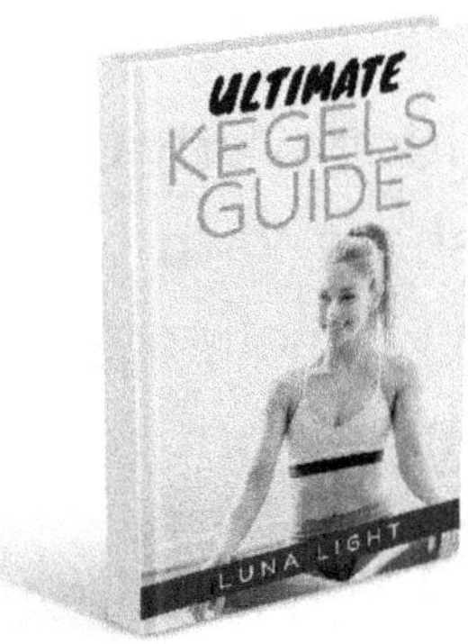

Kegels work for men and women and can help improve your pelvic floor tone, enhance your sex life, and develop your core for better posture. You may have heard of Kegels before... but unfortunately, there is widespread misinformation about hold time, the number of repetitions, and how to actually do the contractions that do more harm than good.

When done right, Kegels are a powerful way to feel stronger and enhance your sex life. The Kegels exercise we created comes directly from Tim Sawyer, a top physical therapist who worked with doctors at Stanford University[*] to develop rehabilitation programs. All you have to do is go to wallpilates.org to download it for free. Alternatively, scan the QR code below:

---

[*]     Dr. Wise and Dr. Anderson authored *A Headache in the Pelvis: A New Understanding and Treatment for Chronic Pelvic Pain Syndromes* (Harmony: 2018) and consulted Tim as the main physical therapist for their treatments.

# **Nutrition** & Balance

*"Let food be thy medicine and medicine be thy food."*
*— Hippocrates*

I am not an expert on giving nutritional advice; however, there is one thing I've studied in depth that I'd like to share with you if you're open to it. This is my observation from years of working with clients on the diet plans that accompany their physical therapy sessions at home and at the gym.

It's not about eating less (reducing caloric intake). It's about having an average intake (eating normally) in a healthy combination that assists in our muscle growth. If you're unsure of what your daily calorie intake should be, just go to Google and search for "calorie calculator" and input your age, activity level, weight, and health goals. (On average, at age 70 for females, the average BMR requires 1,300 to 1,700 calories a day.) You can also use ChatGPT and simply ask, "I am 62, 180 lb., relatively active; what should be my daily calorie intake?"

Rather than calorie counting, we want to achieve the right balance of nutrition in our food. I know it's hard to go from a regular diet to eating completely healthy, so here are two plans: one that's scientifically backed as the "longevity diet" and another diet that is more reasonable for the average person living in a Westernized country.

The **Longevity Diet** is mainly a plant-based diet:

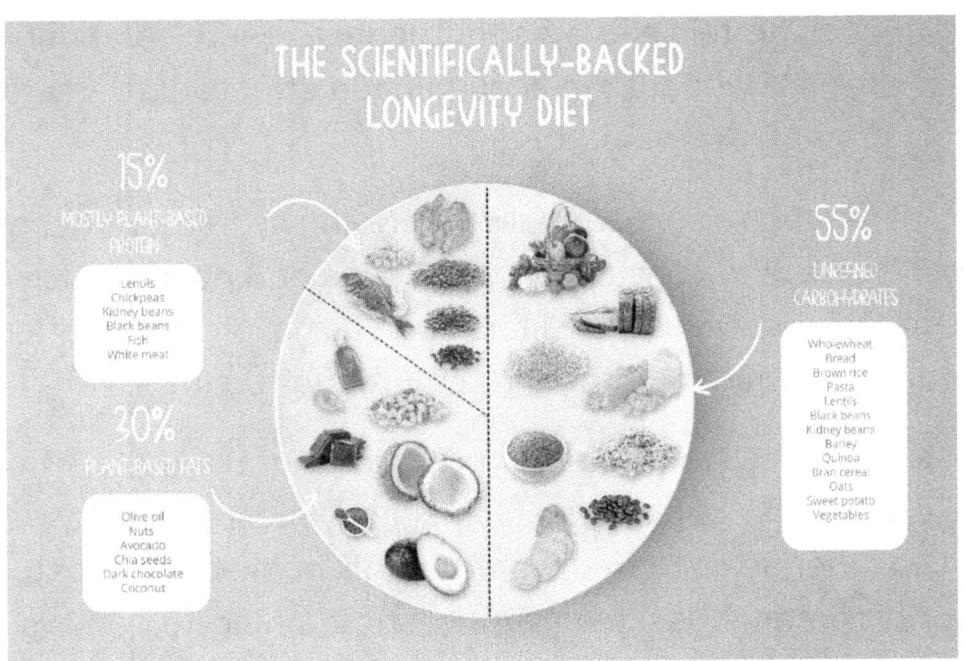



It may look hard at first, but once you learn how to make delicious meals using these ingredients, your whole body just feels lighter all the time. These days, I consume mostly a longevity diet with occasional meat intake.

If this looks too hard for you, don't worry. There's another solution.

A less rigorous **Balanced Diet** includes meat, but at a reasonable 25 percent:

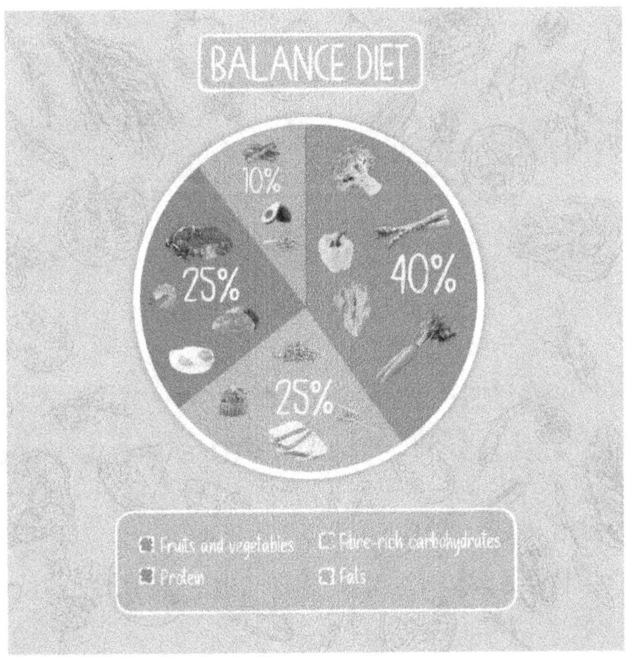

This gives us enough protein and other nutrients to energize us during workouts and build muscle mass without the accumulated effects of overeating red meat as we age.[*]

Remember that nutrition also means always staying hydrated. A general guideline for daily water intake is to consume about 8 cups of 8 ounces each of water per day, which is roughly equivalent to 2 liters or half a gallon. This is often referred to as the **"8x8 rule,"** invented by nutritionist Dr. Fredrick J. Stare.

Being consistent on a balanced diet at your caloric intake levels, when combined with the exercises in this book, is the fastest and safest way to lose weight while gaining the two other goals from the start of this book: better posture and more strength. Our program is designed for holistic training to achieve these three goals at once:

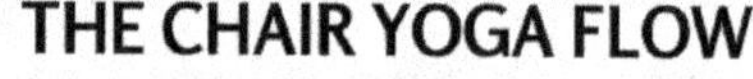


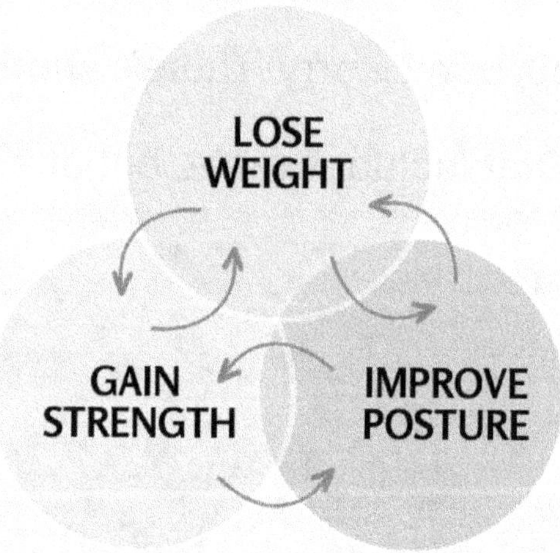


As you gain strength, the additional muscle strength will help you sustain the weight of your body and maintain better posture throughout the day.

As your posture improves, you can perform these exercises to a greater degree of flexibility and experience even more exercise gains.

---

[*]    There are multiple peer-reviewed studies on the effects of red meat on health. See Valter Longo's, *The Longevity Diet,* (Avery, 2018).

As you get better posture and gain strength, you can now work out with greater intensity and more efficient form, thereby burning more calories and losing more weight.

As you lose weight, you are able to stand in a more balanced way and distribute weight more evenly from the top of your head down to your spine and down to your feet on the ground.

All this is happening as your new balanced diet plan gives you the energy to achieve these goals, all while feeling great.

Everything is connected.

# How Chair Yoga Can Help You

*"Yoga is the journey of the self, through the self, to the self."*
— *The Bhagavad Gita*

Chair yoga provides a solution for us to gain strength and mobility while minimizing the chance of injury by using the stabilizing force of the chair. You can do it anytime you're sitting down in the comfort of your own home. You can combine it with other forms of exercise or just do it once a day for fifteen minutes.

| Why Chair Yoga? | Chair Yoga | Other Training Forms |
|---|---|---|
| Injury Risk | Low impact, less chance of inflammation. Stable. | Need resting days, possibility of overtraining and injuring or straining muscles. |
| Accessibility | People with disabilities, injuries, mobility issues, and seniors can still do all exercises safely. | For those with mobility issues, intense weight training routines can be dangerous and set you back more. |
| Intensity | Loving the feeling instead of "forcing it." Less burn out. | Pushing to the limit. |
| Fat Burn | Can still get a good workout and sweat even if mobility is limited. | Can feel exhausting or overtrained. Can't train if limited mobility. |
| Feeling | Feels like you're moving at your own pace, instead of under pressure or "competing." | Feels really sore after, feels fast and rushed. |
| Results | More tone, strength, and spinal alignment using stability of chair. Holistic and accessible. | Isolates specific muscles. Can become muscular but at the expense of holistic health. |

When compared to other forms of exercise, chair yoga is safer and more convenient for seniors, rehabilitation clients, those with mobility issues, or anyone who just wants to start out slowly and comfortably.

The chair allows us to gain all these advantages without any cost.

# **What You Need** to Start



The 28-day program in this book is a guide to help you move at your own pace. It's not a race. To begin...you'll need:

1. **A sturdy chair:** It helps if your chair has four legs and is sturdy. Make sure it can sustain your weight when you lean on it, even if you push heavily. Avoid heavy, immovable chairs, chairs with no back support, and rocking chairs. We're looking for a standard, sturdy, and moveable chair.

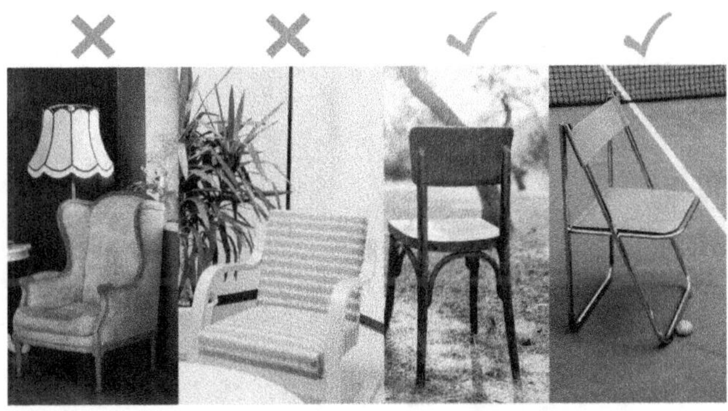

2. **A pillow, a yoga block, or a rolled-up towel** can help you soften the seat and assist as an anchor in certain exercises. This is optional.

3. **Clear space:** Ensure the area around the wall is free from obstacles, slippery rugs, glass, or loose items that could lead to trips or falls.

4. **Footwear and attire:** Wear appropriate, nonslip footwear if you prefer. Chair yoga is very effective barefoot. Comfortable, form-fitting attire can help you move freely without getting tangled or caught.

5. **Water bottle:** Drink plenty of water before, during, and after your exercise session to prevent muscle cramps and promote recovery. I always prepare a water bottle before a workout so I stay hydrated no matter what.

When exercising, if you feel like you're pushing too hard... it's okay to rest and then start again slowly. Consistency is more important than "going hard." My mentor once told me: "Being extraordinary is simply performing ordinary things consistently over a period of time."

So go at your own pace. This isn't a race... there's no competition here. Think of it as playing with your own "limitations" and expanding them beyond your current comfort zone.

# **How To** Breathe (Important!)

*"Breathing is the first act of life and the last. Our very life depends on it. Since we cannot live without breathing, it is tragically deplorable to contemplate the millions and millions who have never mastered the art of correct breathing."*
— Joseph Pilates, inventor of Pilates*

The most important thing to remember is the coordination of the breath to help the movement of your body.

## Practicing Breathing

Try this out. Inhale through your nose: Taking a deep breath in, aim to expand the ribcage out to the sides, allowing the lungs to fill up with air.

Now exhale through the mouth: Purse your lips as if you're blowing out through a straw and exhale fully, engaging your core muscles and feeling the abdominal wall draw inward.

How does it feel? Pretty good, right? Now, try inhaling and exhaling with your mouth fully to 100 percent limit. Do you feel your chest expanding? Lungs reaching places it hasn't gone before? Good. Now, try inhaling and exhaling with your nose. How does that feel? Chances are your nose feels smooth (more filters for pollution through the nostrils), and using your mouth feels like you have more breathing capacity.

The breath gives us so much untapped power. Practicing this increases your breathing capacity and your ability to do more movements. To increase my

---

*     Joseph H. Pilates and William J. Miller. *Return to Life Through Contrology,* (Mockingbird Press, 2021).

breathing abilities, I use visualization. When I'm practicing, I'm sitting down on the chair or lying on the floor in the corpse pose. Sometimes, I take the lightning (yoga) pose.

**Corpse pose:**

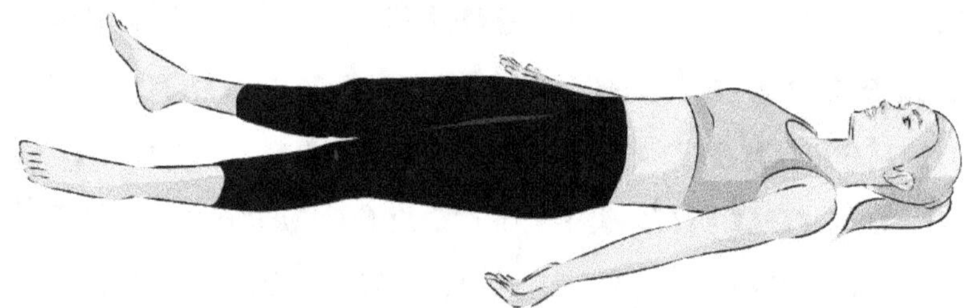

**Lightning pose:**

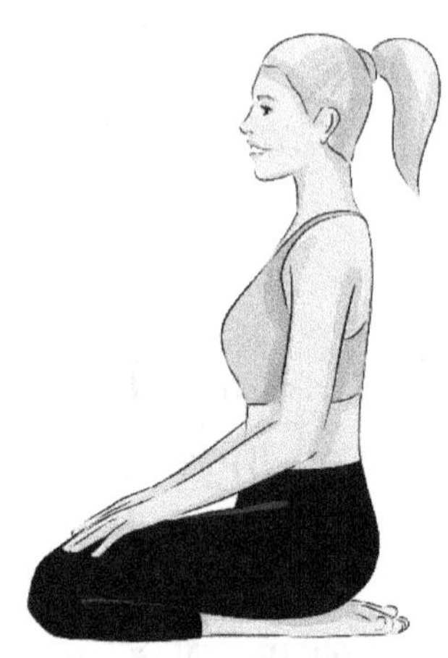

I imagine my rib cage expanding. Then I imagine my abdomen expanding, then my upper back, then my lower back. With each breath, I see if I can expand my lungs and diaphragm in all directions. This practice has improved my breathing capacity significantly after just a few months. Note that if you use your mouth to inhale and exhale, you can expand further with more air and then revert back to nose breathing on subsequent counts. When I first started, I was limited to nose breathing, which I was told is healthier (which is true), but when my teacher taught me to breathe in using my mouth, I suddenly was able to expand my chest and lungs, and I realized I was severely limited by years of nose breathing to the point where my chest wasn't even moving and my air intake was low!

Do ten minutes of this every morning and see how your breathing capacity changes in just a few short weeks.

## A Sure Way to Feel Calm

The 4-7-8 technique, also known as the "relaxing breath," is a simple breathing exercise developed by Dr. Andrew Weil. It's inspired by an ancient yogic technique called *pranayama,* which involves the regulation of breath to enhance physical and mental well-being.

The 4-7-8 technique is designed to act as a natural tranquilizer for the nervous system, so it's great at the end of a workout. In fact, I use it whenever I feel rushed or stressed outside the gym.

**4-7-8 Steps:**

1. Inhale quietly through the nose for a count of four.

2. Hold your breath for a count of seven.

3. Exhale completely through the mouth, making a whoosh sound, for a count of eight.

This is one breath cycle. Aim to complete this cycle for four breaths while you relax.

## Box Breathing

Box breathing, also known as square breathing, is a relaxation and stress reduction technique that has been utilized in various practices, including yoga, meditation, and tactical settings in the military. The best part about this is that it's easy to remember: Four seconds in, four seconds hold, four seconds out, four seconds hold.

Box breathing has been used to help soldiers and law enforcement personnel manage stress and anxiety and maintain focus in high-pressure situations. Special operations units and tactical training programs often incorporate this breathing technique as a means to enhance performance and cognitive control.

The technique itself—employing a pattern of controlled breaths in a four-part sequence—has deep roots in ancient practices, especially in disciplines such as yoga and meditation. Pranayama, the yogic practice of breath control, features various breathing exercises, some of which resemble the box breathing technique. These ancient practices aim to regulate and control the breath to improve physical, mental, and emotional well-being. Here are the practice instructions:

**Breathing Pattern:** Follow this sequence for each breath phase:

- **Inhale (4 seconds):** Breathe in slowly and deeply through your nose for a count of four seconds. Feel your lungs expanding as you do so.

- **Hold (4 seconds):** Once you've inhaled fully, hold your breath for four seconds. Be comfortable, and don't strain yourself.

- **Exhale (4 seconds):** Slowly exhale through your mouth for a count of four seconds. Release the air completely from your lungs.

- **Hold (4 seconds):** After exhaling, hold your breath again for another four seconds before starting the cycle again.

- **Repeat** for as long as you need to feel calm.

# **Tai Chi** and Pilates

One of the main philosophies in tai chi is instead of fighting against "it" (life, your muscles, your body limitations), adapt and evolve with it.

Tai chi movements follow the breath and use the natural flow of chi to guide slow, comfortable movements. If you ever get a chance to walk by a group of elders doing tai chi in the morning, you can sense their calm energy and vibrancy.

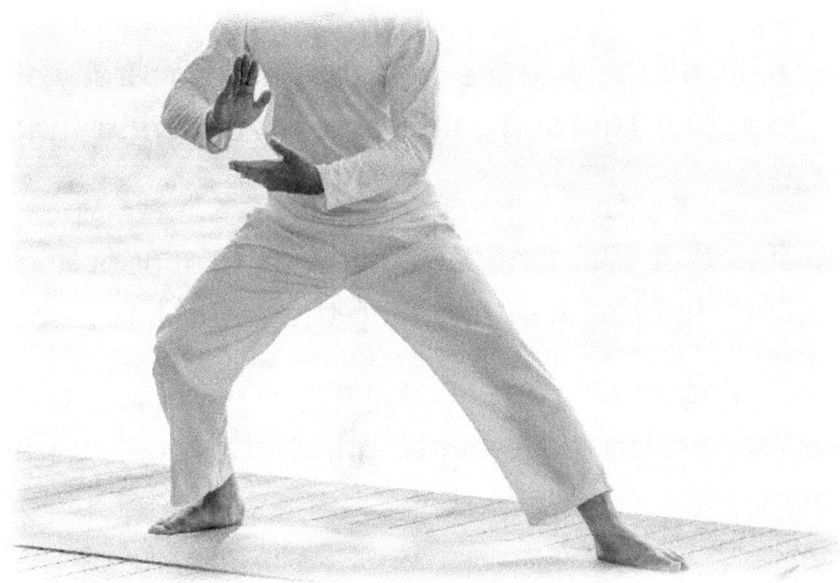

In *Caged Lion,* John Howard Steel talks about "Pilates [as] a system of coordinated movement, concentration, and breathing that fully absorbs the actor in what he or she is doing, adds grace and efficiency to daily life, relieves stress, increases circulation, augments self-esteem, becomes a habit, and most importantly is fun to do.*" Pilates exercises don't feel like they're going against you or like something you have to conquer. Just look at the calmness of even a more difficult movement:

---

* John Howard Steel. *Caged Lion: Joseph Pilates & His Legacy* (p. 178). (Last Leaf Press, 2020). Kindle Edition.

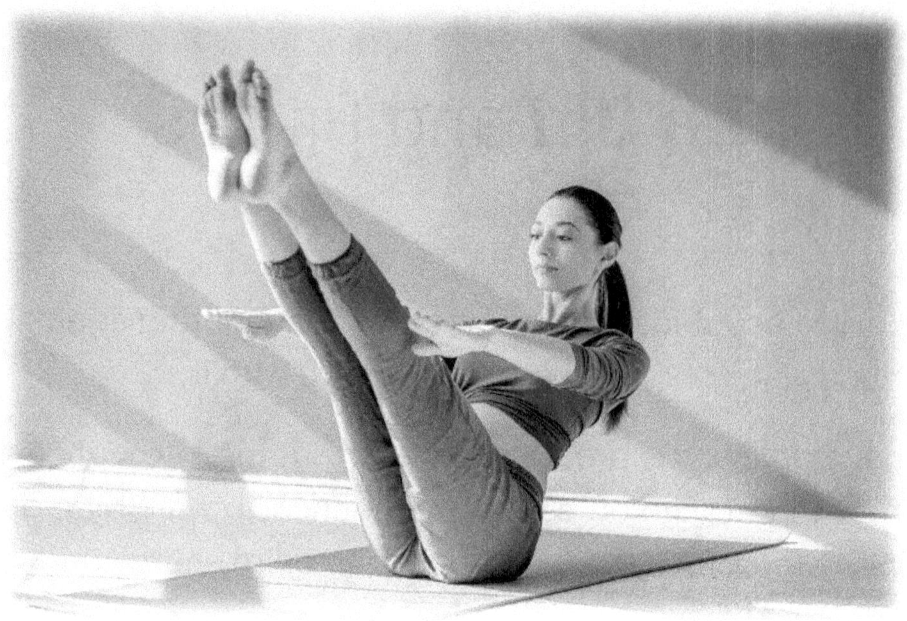

Both Pilates and tai chi emphasize the presence and accuracy of slow moments. By going slow, we're actually getting gains faster by concentrating all the muscles in the movements.

The philosophies of both movements also allow us to accept and adapt to aging, instead of consistently fighting it or resisting the natural signs of it.

As you do the following chair yoga exercises, I invite you to think about the philosophy of slow, controlled movements, guided by your breath and the natural energy flow of your body.

# **The Workout** Plan

This 28-day chair yoga program incorporates warm-ups and balance training first. Then, we focus on a holistic workout program that targets your entire body using cardio training, flexibility training, and strength training.

| DAY | EXERCISE | DAY | EXERCISE |
| --- | --- | --- | --- |
| 1 | Group 1 and 2 | 15 | Group 1 and 2 |
| 2 | Group 1 and 2 | 16 | Group 1 and 2 |
| 3 | Group 1 and 3 | 17 | Group 1, 2, 3 |
| 4 | Group 1 and 3 | 18 | Group 1, 2, 4 |
| 5 | Group 1, 2, 3 | 19 | Group 1, 2, 4 |
| 6 | Break day | 20 | Break day |
| 7 | Group 1 and 2 | 21 | Group 1 and 2 |
| 8 | Group 1, 2, 3 | 22 | Group 1, 2, 3 |
| 9 | Group 1, 2, 3 | 23 | All exercises |
| 10 | Group 1, 2, 4 | 24 | All exercises |
| 11 | Group 1, 2, 4 | 25 | All exercises |
| 12 | Group 1, 2, 4 | 26 | All exercises |
| 13 | Break day | 27 | Break day |
| 14 | Group 1 and 2 | 28 | All exercises |

**Gentle recovery version, if you're mobility-limited or going through rehabilitation:**

- Start with group 1 for the first 1–7 days.

- Do group 1 and 2 for days 7–14.

- Do group 1, 2, and 4 for days 15–21.

- Do group 1 and 3 for days 21–28.

# BALANCE EXERCISES

Every time you start a workout session, begin with these balance awareness exercises.

**This is super important, especially if you are a senior. Please don't skip this.**

Without proper balance awareness, we risk injury, doing the exercises incorrectly, and using bad form. This negates all the work you're putting in!

In addition, doing these balance exercises over time will also help you totally reshape the way you stand, move, and do everything.

You will feel lighter and more free instead of heavy and slow. Maybe pain in certain areas due to repetitive use and misuse will go away. Maybe your movements set feelings free, and you're aware of bad habits and correct them right away. Maybe life starts to flow again.

Try it out and go through this section every time you exercise.

Without stability, bad form can cause injuries and repetitive stress to your whole body. That's why we want to perform all exercises in a stable manner. As you gain stability, everything you do will feel more balanced. We'll call this "balance awareness."

The first step in balance awareness is your feet.

BALANCE CHECK INSTRUCTIONS

1   Stand straight in front of a mirror facing the wall.

2   Feel the alignment of both your feet. Are they properly aligned, or is one foot in front of the other? Are your toes pointed forward with a slight outward tilt? This is the natural alignment of the feet:

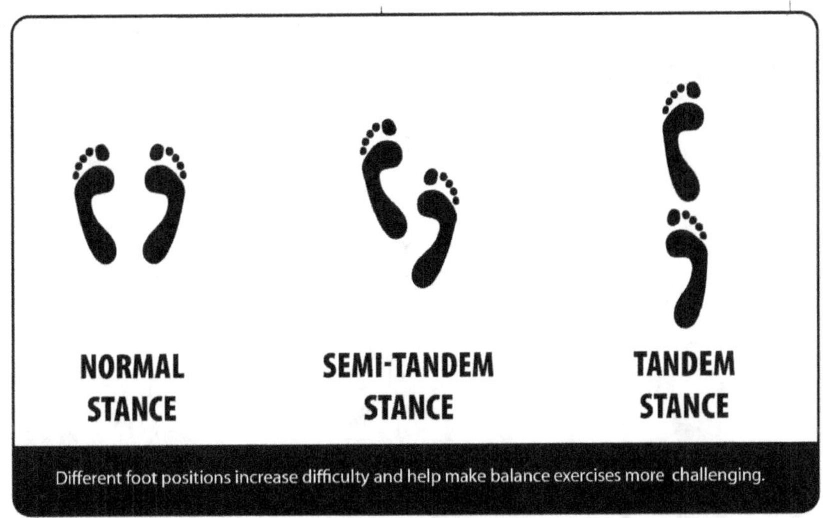


3   Now, feel the weight of your body on your feet. Where is the point of center? Is it toward your toes? Or are you always "on your heels?" Or always "tip-toeing" around? The center of weight should be toward the center of your foot, straight down from the ankles.

4   Stop here, take a breath, and feel your weight distribution—it should be balanced fifty-fifty on both feet. Imagine your spine passing down toward your knees and down to your ankles. The image below shows all the alignments you can build awareness around: the head controlled by the neck, the shoulders, the core and hips, your knees, and your feet.

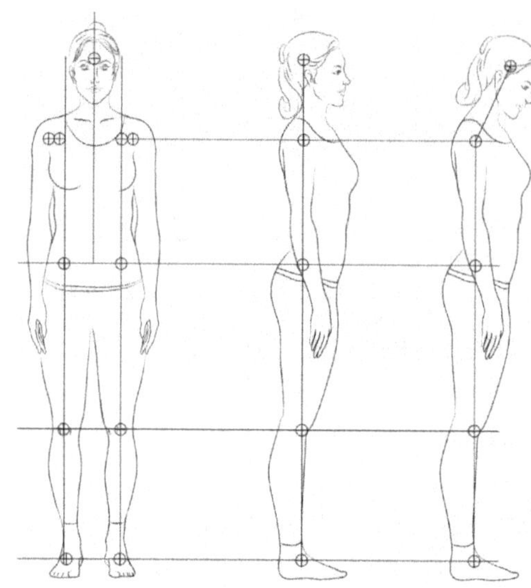

5  Use a mirror and look directly at your alignment from head to toe. Turn sideways and look now. How does your body feel? With your face forward, feel the weight distribution on your feet. Take three breaths here and just feel your body. Imagine a smooth line that goes from the top of your head down your spine and through your feet into the ground. Here are some examples of common dysfunctions:

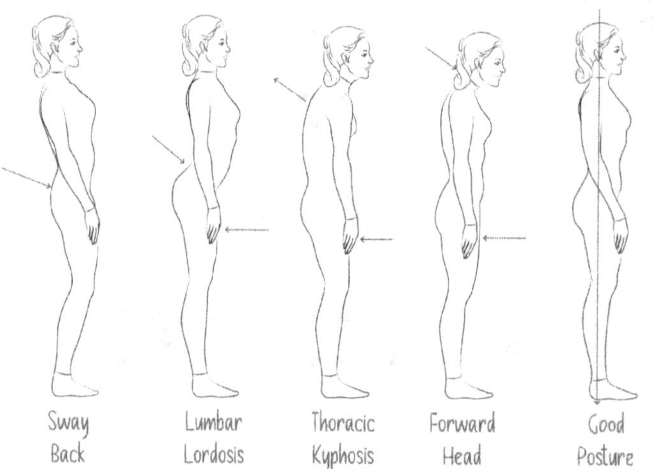


Don't worry about getting it 100 percent right. Just being aware of this will increase your ability to correct any postural issues over time. This exercise trains your mind to become aware of your body's alignment as you go about your day.

The Alexander technique is a method that focuses on improving posture, movement, and overall physical coordination. Developed by F. Matthias Alexander in the 1890s, it is often used to alleviate chronic pain, improve posture, and enhance body awareness.

In this exercise, we're going to use the chair for balance as I help you find the right posture.

Many people are unaware that they have bad posture, which, over time, leads to limited mobility, pain, and other health problems.

## SITTING INSTRUCTIONS

1  Using the chair as support if you feel unbalanced, feel your head, spine, and legs as you sit down. Do you feel like your whole body is aligned, or is there an uneven distribution of weight?

2  Now, try sitting down. Does your sitting down look more like the image on the left or the right below?

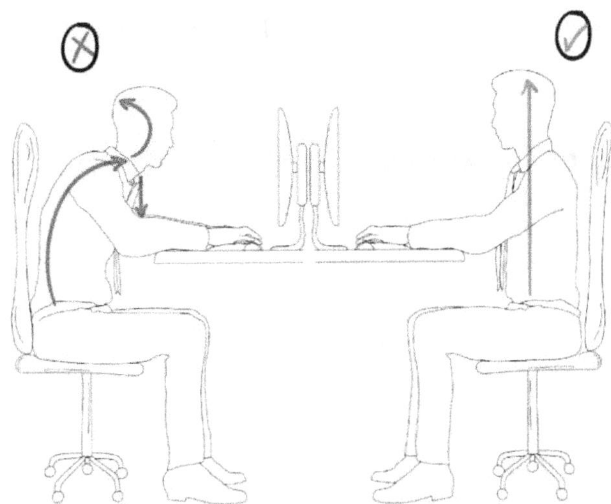

3  Try standing and sitting down three times. Each time, build awareness of how your body is moving. You may even do it in front of a bedroom mirror and watch your posture carefully.

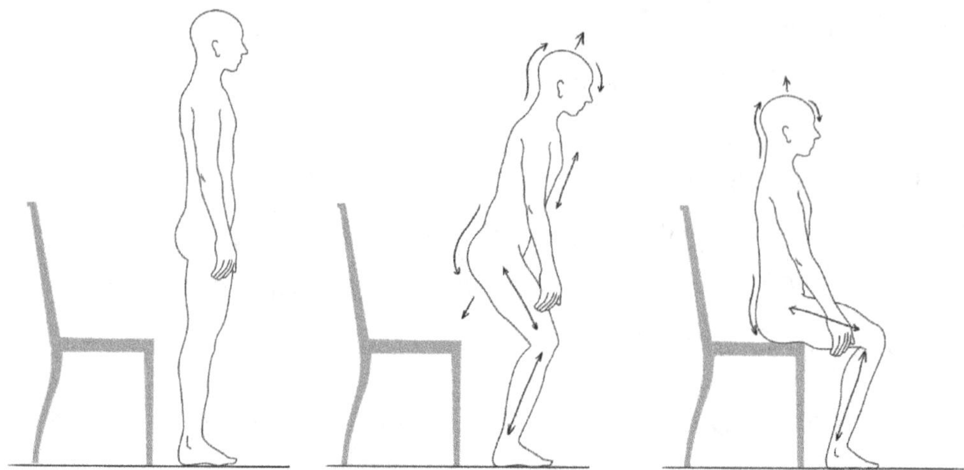

4   Now, let's try sitting down using these instructions. To sit down in a chair, we lower the trunk so that the bottom part of the pelvis or your "sit bones" can rest on the chair. Note: Your sit bones are the two bony prominences at the bottom of the pelvis that you can feel when you sit down.

5   Bend the hips, knees, and ankles so your hips feel like they are moving backward.

6   Lower your hips to the chair by flexing further, bringing your sit bones into contact with the chair, with the weight of the hips still mainly over the feet.

7   Once the sit bones are on the chair, straighten your spine so that the weight of your pelvic area is directly over the sit bones and you are sitting fully upright.

**Notice how this feels compared to how you usually sit.**

Now, stand up next to the chair and explore your standing posture. Don't worry. The chair is there to support you if you lose balance or need a rest.

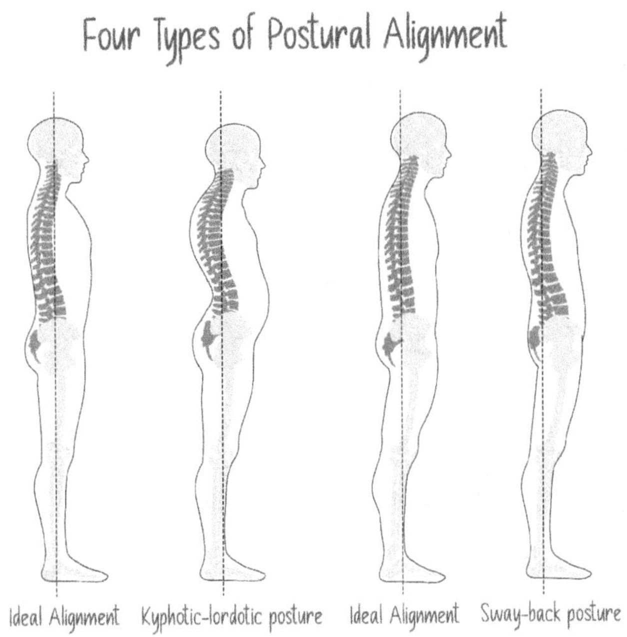



The following standing instructions are from my mentor, a 24-year master of the Alexander technique on how to stand.

STANDING INSTRUCTIONS

Standing up straight, do the following steps:

## A. The first step is "Inhibition."

Pausing. Before each movement, as well as before "directing," pause. Inhibit your tendency to react immediately to your habitual unnecessary tensions.

## B. The Five Directions

1. Neck free

2. Head forward and up

3. Back lengthening and widening

4. Upper arms away from each other

5. Knees forward and away from each other

**Or, simply by using intention, your body will auto-respond:**

1. "I choose to allow my neck to release," or "I choose to allow my neck to soften," or "to be free" or "to unlock."

2. "I choose to allow my head to release forward and upward," or "I choose to allow an inner nodding of my head."

3. "I choose to allow my back to lengthen and widen, springing from my feet through the top of my head and expanding."

4. "I choose to allow the upper parts of my arms to go away from each other."

5. "I choose to allow my knees to go forward away from my hip joints and away from each other."

Here is how you practice the first two directions:

**1) "I want" (or "I choose") to allow my neck to release."**

With that intention, you ask the suboccipital muscles to unclench.

**(So that my head can go forward and up.)**

**2) "I want" (or "I choose") to allow my head to release forward and up."**

I want my head to be free to release into a nod and away from my feet.

In short: **Neck free, head forward and up.**

**Remember to use intention, not "doing."**

This practice will help you:

- Develop your body awareness and ability to be in the present moment.

- Make you aware of excess tension in your suboccipital area and consequently of tensions in your whole body.

- Diminish the stress placed on your neck and spine.

- Release your antigravity mechanism and ease up your whole body.

- Develop your ability to help yourself to reach, at will, your optimal state of ease.

- Help you prevent injuries.

<u>When to practice:</u>

Start with situations in which your mind is free to focus on yourself:

- Walking from one room to the next

- Walking from your office to your car

- Hiking

- Standing in line waiting at a counter

- Standing while talking on the phone

- Sitting while being on hold on the phone

For example, next time, notice how you use your phone, and if you're reading the Kindle version of this book, this is a good opportunity to ask: Are you overextending your neck to look down? In the graphic below, the posture in the middle is less stressful for the body than the one on the right, where the neck and hand are inefficiently extended:

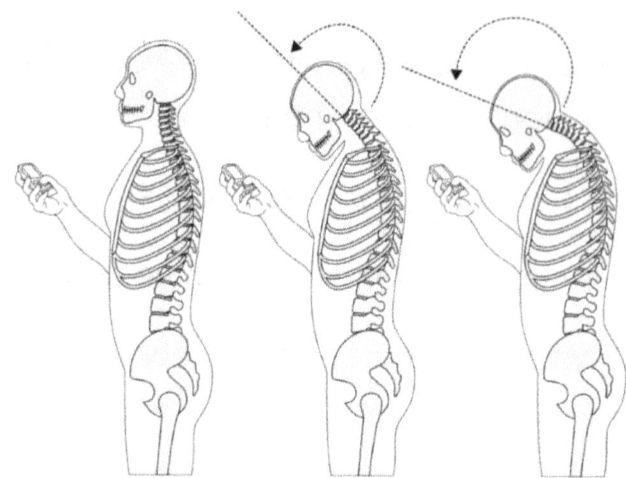

With practice, experiment in more complex situations like interacting with others or during strenuous activities involving physical effort, such as bending or lifting.

***Warning: Do not "try" to make anything happen. Avoid engaging muscles in the attempt to achieve a "good" position of your head. Use the power of your intention to allow a release to happen.***

Whatever position your head is in (including tilting your head backward in order to look up), you need an attitude of readiness to nod a "yes" (the "forward" direction) while you hold an intention for your head to rise upward, away from the floor.

(The "up" direction becomes "outward" direction if your body is not vertical as in lying down or bending from standing to sitting. It goes away from the base of your spine in any position.)

These first two directions are simple yet require repeated practice to identify, stop, and prevent the habits caused by a lifetime of challenges.

The next three directions integrating the whole body will be:

**I want to allow my whole body to expand from my feet or my sit bones.**

**I want to allow my knees to go forward and away from each other.**

**I want to allow my shoulders to move away from each other.**

Alexander used to say about the five directions: "One after the other, all at the same time." The first two directions make it possible for the whole body to expand, and at the same time, you need to be grounded for the head to be totally free to release forward and up.

I highly recommend that if you sense you have a serious postural issue, seek out a licensed Alexander technique teacher and have them guide you for a few sessions. You can find a full official list at alexandertechnique.com. Once you have "felt" the proper posture from a great teacher, return to this book to continue to the exercises.

Once you "feel" what correct posture is like, you'll want to achieve that state of freedom again and again, which is the greatest motivator.

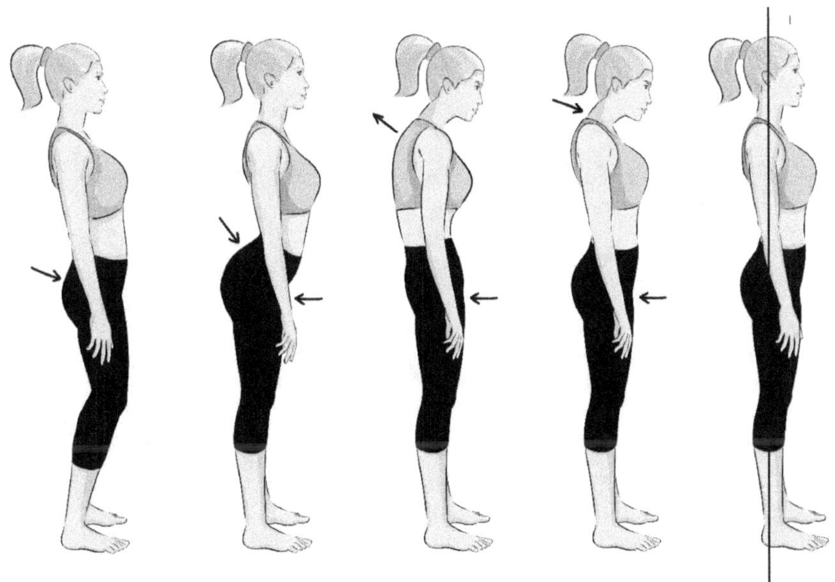

For me, when I was in constant chronic pain, after an adjustment or guidance from my Alexander technique teacher, I would always be pain-free for a few hours. Let's just say pain is a great motivator to learn!

This exercise is optional; it usually takes about ten minutes. But if you do it consistently, it will continue to improve your posture and make it into an unconscious habit. People may even start complimenting you on your posture and the way you move!

You can find great books on the Alexander technique on Amazon, but if this chapter interests you, I highly recommend finding a certified teacher and FEEL the difference in your body. In the US, that's https://www.amsatonline.org/. All the legit certified instructors require the standard 1,600 hours of training over three years!

This is an Alexander technique designed to build spinal awareness.

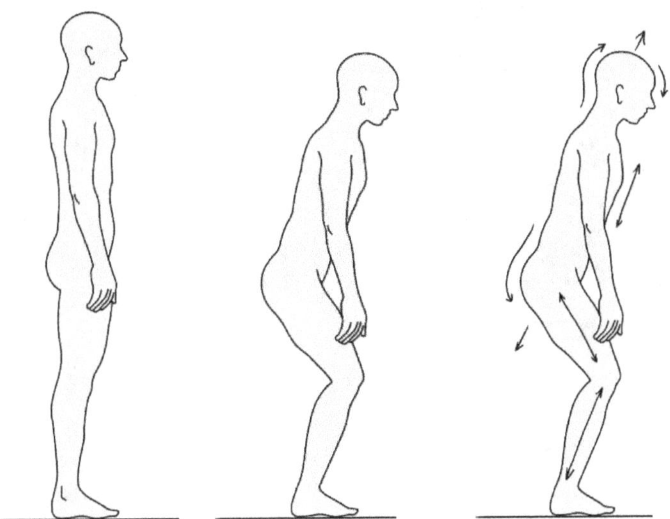

THE MONKEY INSTRUCTIONS

1. You're in a standing position. Come to your full height by allowing your neck to release to let your head go forward and up and your back to lengthen.

2. Now, think of releasing your buttocks muscles outward and downward as you bend your knees.

3. As your butt draws down and its muscles let go, think of releasing the front of your hip joints, behind your knees, and the front of your ankles. I think of this as my head leading the spine to lengthen my lower legs.

4. Allow your knees to release from your lower back, so now you're bending a bit forward but still with a straight spine. This should give you much more freedom and release in your thighs, and you will feel strength in your lower back and pelvic area. Basically, you're lengthening your back while bending your knees. This is great for lower back pain. Hang out here for a few seconds.

5. Using your leg muscles and hip muscles, push yourself back to standing. Try doing three monkeys slowly with full body awareness.

Oftentimes, prolonged body misalignment creates shortening of the muscles in the body. This creates postural dysfunctions leading to hip and back pain, shoulder pain, and head and neck pain. The inefficiencies of movement over time add unnecessary stress to your muscles and joints.

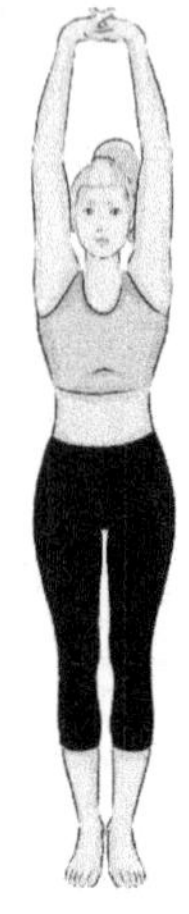

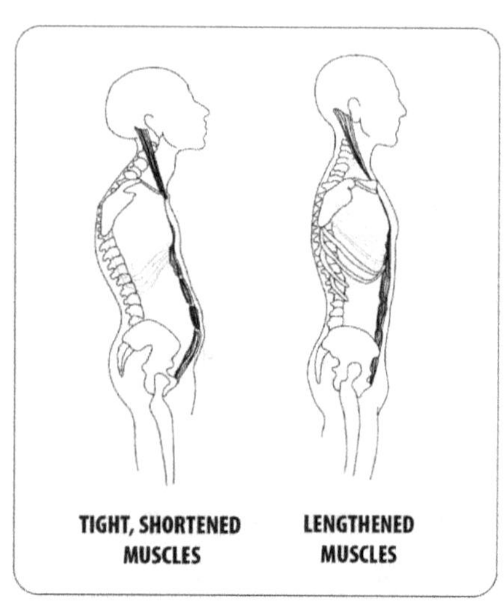



We are going to do a stretch that lengthens your whole body. It's called a torso stretch in yoga, except we're going to do this with the awareness of the whole spine.

1. Standing straight, raise your hands upward.

2. Interlock your fingers, and now see how far up you can go.

3. Go as far as you can; on tiptoe is fine as you can reach further.

4. Tilt your head upward and a little backward, and stretch as far as you can. Stay here for five breaths.

5. Now release your hands and return to a normal standing position.

6. Repeat this three times.

**Tips:**

- Be aware of your spine alignment as you do this.

- Don't lock your knees. Keep them slightly bent and fluid.

# Hip Circles

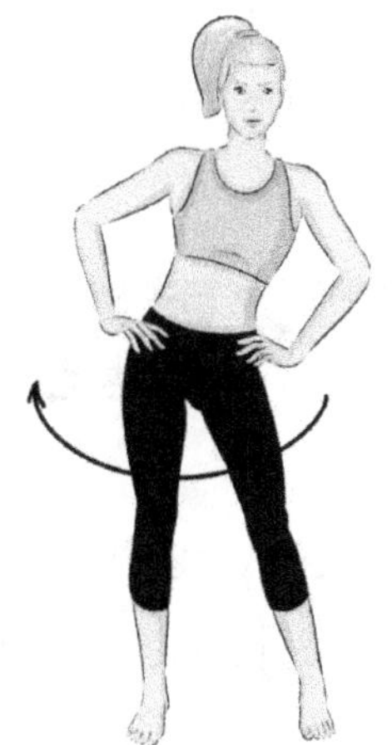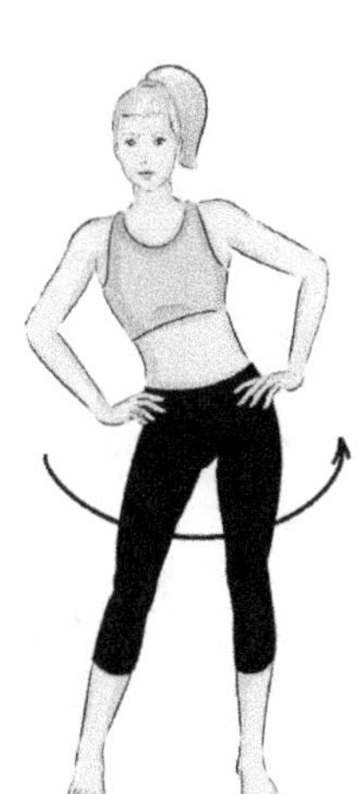

1 Stand with your feet hip-width apart and place your hands on your hips.

2 Rotate your hips outward (clockwise), keeping the upper body stable. Circle as far as you can while maintaining stability. Perform 10 circles.

3 Now rotate your hips inward (anticlockwise), keeping the upper body stable. Circle as far as you can while maintaining stability. Perform 10 circles.

**Tips:**

- Breathe steadily throughout the exercise.

- When doing this, feel your hips align with the spine. Do they feel intact or out of place? This is a great exercise to help you sense any posture issues with your hips.

# WARM-UP EXERCISES

A proper warm-up gently activates your muscles. It gets the blood flowing and improves your joint lubrication. All this prevents potential injuries.

When I first started, I thought warm-ups were for "weak" people and that I would just "skip to the good part." Not good. I got injured, and nowadays, I always warm up.

Think of these warm-ups as a fun game! They are easy, and they feel great.

# Seated Chest Claps

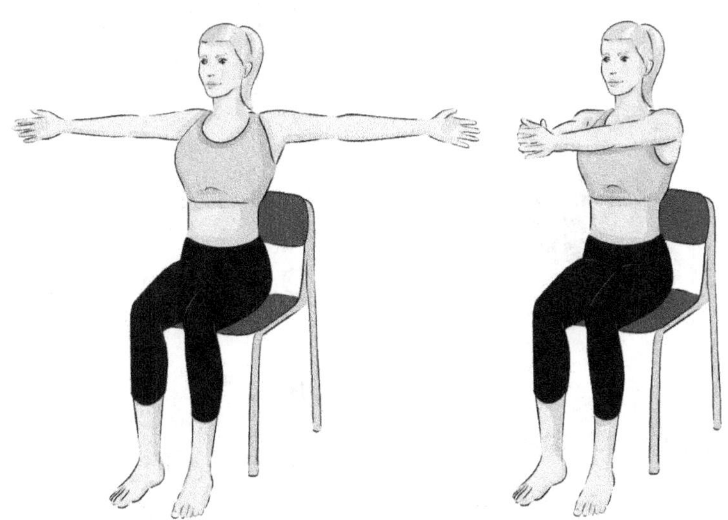

1. Sit down on a chair or on the ground with your back straight and chest up.

2. Place your hands outward with your feet comfortably apart.

3. Bring your hands together in front of your chest, then return to the starting position.

4. Go at your own pace. Speed up for faster cardio and slow down for more control. Experiment with what feels good to you.

5. Perform fifteen chest claps, keeping your core engaged.

**Tips:**

- Try doing this super-slow at first to get the proper form and breathing right.

- After you have the movement down, try going faster to see if you can get a sweat going. This super-fun movement is enjoyable first thing in the morning.

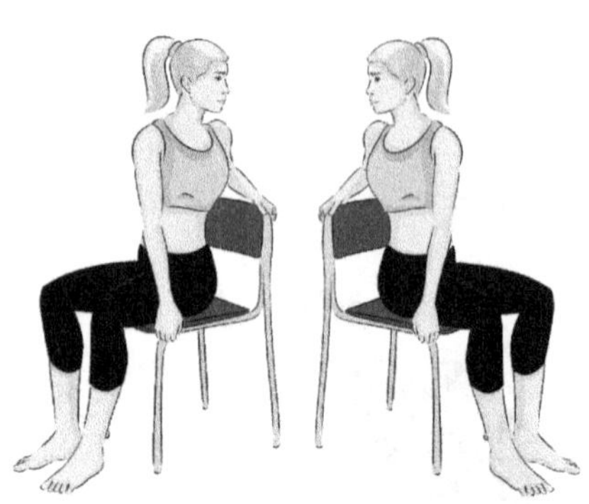

spine, turn backward as far as you comfortably can.

3  Now return to center and turn to the other side.

4  Do 20 reps of 10 on each side.

**Tips:**

Don't sacrifice the turn distance for bad form or by twisting and tightening your core or your spine. Instead, gain length by visualizing extending your spine.

1  Sit down on a chair or on the ground with your back straight and your chest up.

2  Place your arm on the backrest of the chair and, as you lengthen your

## Chair Side Stretch

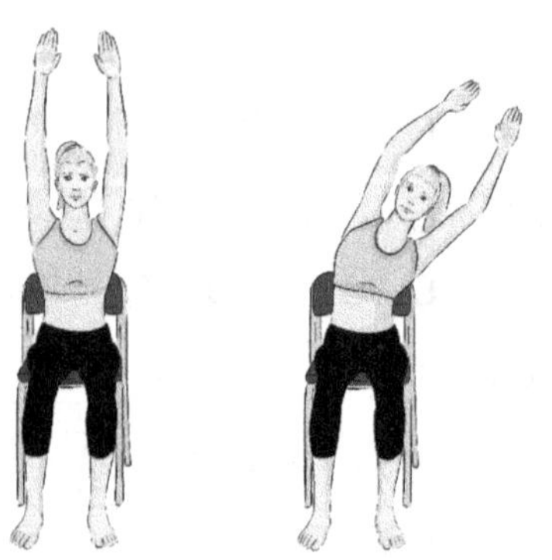

2  Take a few breaths and lengthen your spine. As you do, lean to the right with your hands leading.

3  Now return to center and turn to the other side.

4  Perform twenty reps of ten on each side.

**Tips:**

Don't sacrifice the leaning distance by tightening muscles. Gain mobility by lengthening your muscles.

1  Sit up straight on a chair with your feet flat on the floor and your hands raised high up in the air.

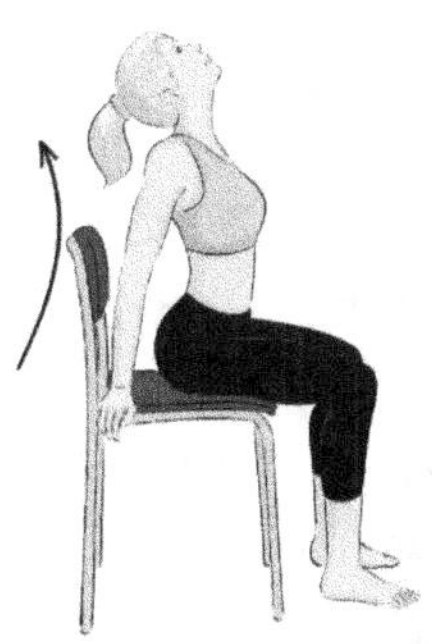

1. Sit halfway to the edge and straight up on a chair with your feet flat on the floor. Place your hands behind you firmly on the seat.

2. As you inhale, lengthen your spine and lift your chest. Arch your back and tilt your head upward and backward as far as you can.

3. As you exhale, slowly return to a normal sitting position.

4. Do ten reps.

**Tips:**

Don't sit too close to the edge as it's dangerous. Find the center and scoot just enough to place your hands on the chair firmly.

## Chair Downward Stretch

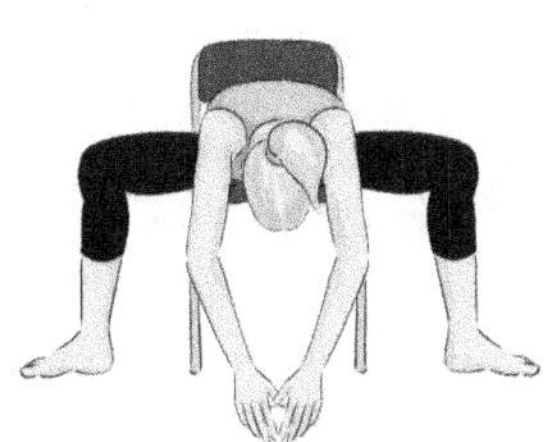

1. Sit up straight on a chair with your legs as widely extended as possible.

2. Inhale a deep breath. As you exhale, bend forward with your hands as far down as you can.

3. Repeat five times. Each time you extend down, try to go a little further.

**Tips:**

- Avoid sitting or sitting too close to the chair's edge.

- If you're super-flexible and can touch the ground, see if you can bring your elbows to the ground.

# Chair Arm Circle

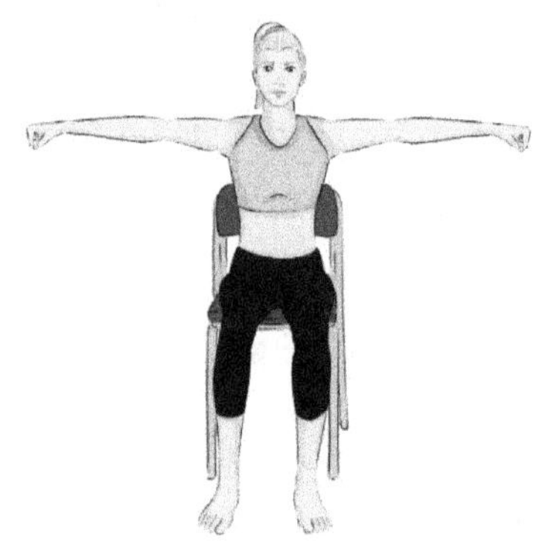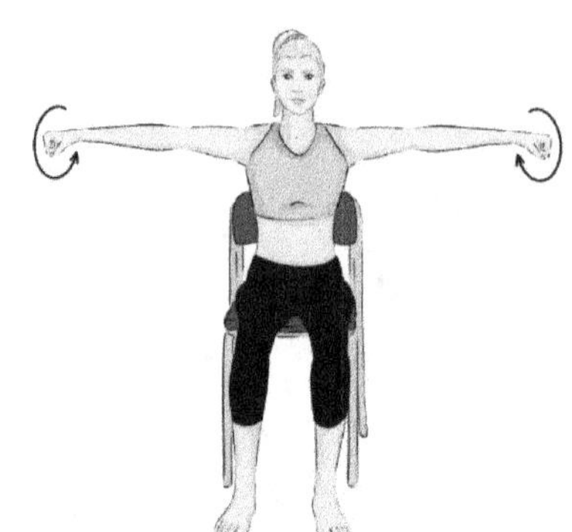

1. Sit up straight on a chair with your feet flat on the floor.

2. Extend your arms straight out to the sides, parallel to the floor.

3. Begin making small circular motions with your arms, like you're drawing circles with your hands. You can use an open-handed palm or your fists.

4. Continue the circular motions for ten seconds.

5. Now, go in the other direction for ten seconds.

**Tips:**

- Maintain slow and controlled movements to avoid straining your shoulders.

- Gradually increase the size of the circles as you feel comfortable.

# CARDIO EXERCISES

There are many benefits to cardiovascular exercise, from improved metabolism to improved lung capacity and improved sleep... the list goes on.

If you've heard the term "Yoga Body," it's because the following exercises not only use cardio to burn calories, they also strengthen and tone your muscle groups at the same time so you end up looking amazing.

Our main goal is not weight loss. It's just a byproduct of this form of exercise. You see... we are using low-impact exercises designed to strengthen muscles, improve postural alignment, and enhance flexibility.

So not only will you lose weight if you do these exercises consistently while having a balanced diet... you'll feel stronger, more flexible, and move with a more aligned posture. Is that motivating enough for you?

Let's get started!

# Chair Leg Extension

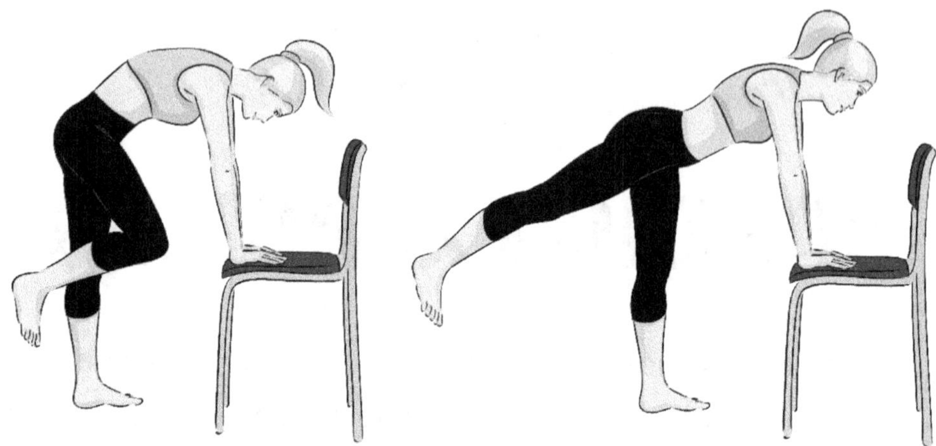

1 Place your hands on the sides of the chair seat for stability.

2 Lift one leg off the ground, then extend it fully behind you.

3 Hold your leg extended for three seconds.

4 Now, return your leg back to the starting position slowly. It's still lifted from the ground.

5 Repeat this ten times.

6 Change legs and repeat this extension ten times.

7 Breathe naturally as you perform the leg extensions.

**Tips:**

- Keep your back straight, engage your core, and maintain control throughout the exercise.

- You can speed up or increase reps as you become more familiar with this exercise.

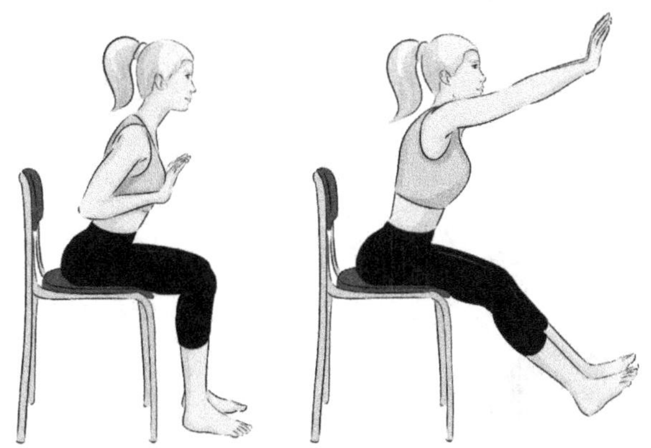

2  Extend your hands upward and your feet forward at the same time at about a 45-degree angle upward and downward, respectively.

3  Come back to the original position and repeat fifteen times.

**Tips:**

Keep your spine straight as you do this.

1  Sit in a chair leaning forward with your hands in front of your chest.

## Sitting Duck Pose

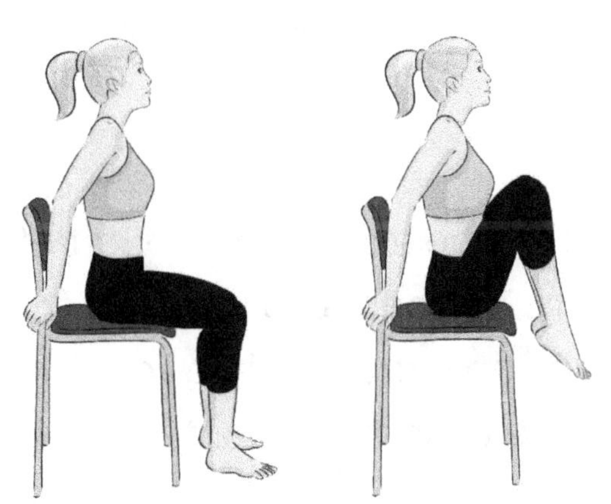

3  Hold for up to three seconds. Try to breathe and maintain balance.

4  Return your feet to the ground.

5  Repeat this ten times.

**Tips:**

You can increase the hold for up to five seconds as you get stronger.

1  Begin by sitting and placing your hands on the back of the chair for stability.

2  As you exhale, bend your knees and lift your legs. Keep your weight on your sit bones.

# Torso Twist

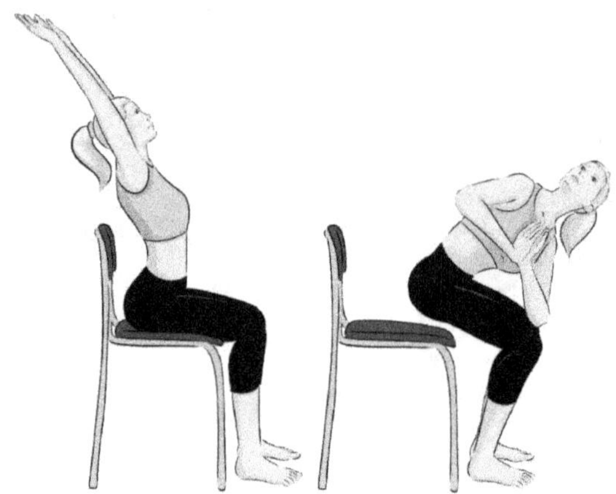

1. Sit upright in a sturdy chair with your feet flat on the ground.

2. Reach upward and backward with your hands, arching your arms for a good stretch.

3. Bring your arms downward all the way and turn to the right, placing your elbow between or close to your knees. Hold here for three seconds as you take deep breaths.

4. Reach upward again for a good stretch, and this time, come down, turning left as you place your elbows between or close to your knees.

5. Repeat the movement, switching from left to right and again up to a total of ten times (five on each side).

**Tips:**

Move on the exhale for a burst of energy. You can also move on the inhale and exhale to use your breath to guide your movements.

# Chair Warrior Pose

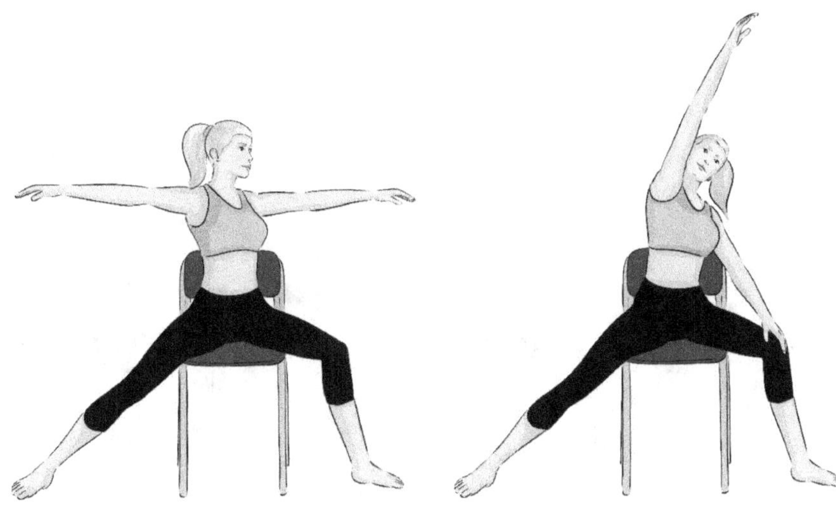

1. Start in a sitting position with your feet three to four feet apart with the chair in the middle as a stabilizer.

2. Turn your left foot out while your right foot straightens outward.

3. Extend your arms out to the sides.

4. Bend your left knee to a 90-degree angle while keeping your right leg straight.

5. Keep your torso facing forward and gaze over your left hand. Hold the warrior pose here for five seconds.

6. Now, move your right hand upward and to the left as far as you comfortably can. Hold for five seconds.

7. Do this for five reps.

8. Now repeat this for the other side (right foot 90-degree angle, left foot straight).

**Tips:**

As you get stronger, you can do this without the chair.

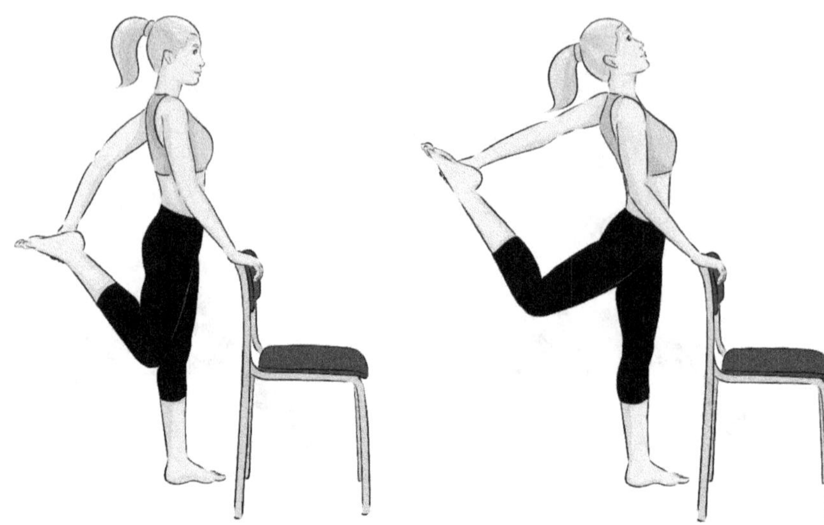

1 Stand behind the chair and use one hand to stabilize yourself.

2 Lift your right foot backward and hold it with your left hand.

3 Extend your legs and spine and lift your leg even further upward and backward. Hold for five seconds, then release.

4 Repeat five times.

5 Now do this for the other side (left foot backward, holding it with your right hand).

6 Repeat five times.

**Tips:**

As you gain increased balance, you can do this without holding onto the chair. You can still stand close to the chair for support in case you lose balance.

# Sitting Jacks

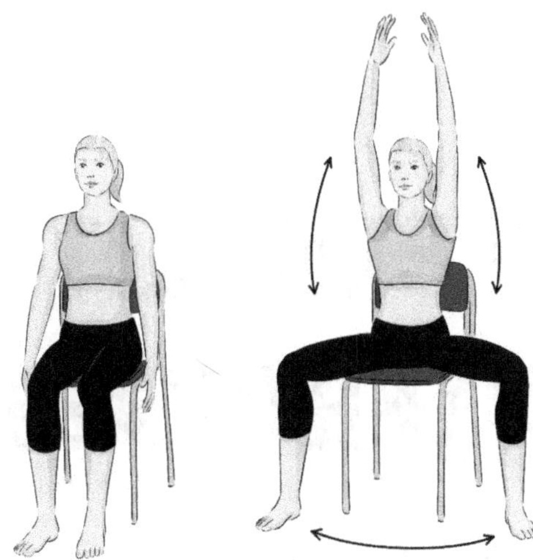

1. Sit on a chair with your feet flat on the floor and your back straight.

2. Start with your feet together and your arms at your sides.

3. In one fluid motion, jump your feet apart and raise your arms overhead, just like a traditional jumping jack, but while remaining seated.

4. Return to the starting position with your feet together and your arms at your sides.

5. Repeat this up to fifteen times. Try to maintain a steady rhythm.

**Tips:**

- You can increase the speed and intensity of this for more cardio and slow it down for more flexibility and control.

- You can increase the reps to thirty as you gain strength and endurance.

# FLEXIBILITY EXERCISES

In Pilates as well as yoga...

Control = Flexibility + Strength

In this section, we are not doing rapid, high-repetition sets but rather performing slower, precise movements with full muscular control. Remember the tai chi and Pilates concepts mentioned earlier? In fact, some Pilates instructors ban the use of the word "exercise" and instead use the word "movement" in their books and trainings.

Why is this important? Because with slow, controlled movements, we are working out our fast-twitch muscle fibers (type II) and slow-twitch muscle fibers (type I) for maximum gains. We also reduce the risk of injury while doing so.

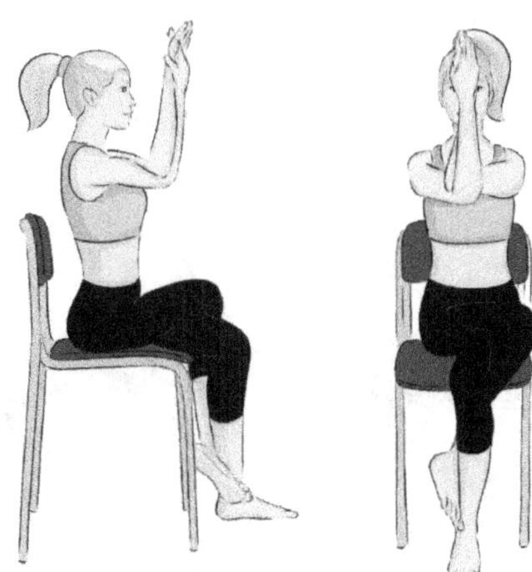

1. Sit on a chair with your feet flat on the floor and your back straight.

2. Lift your right leg and cross it over your left thigh as if you were sitting cross-legged.

3. If possible, tuck your right foot behind your left calf for a deeper stretch.

4. Cross your arms in front of your chest with your right arm under your left.

5. Bend your elbows and bring your palms together if you can. If not, simply touch your opposite shoulders with your hands.

6. Sit up straight and engage your core.

7. Hold the chair eagle pose for fifteen seconds, feeling a stretch in your upper back and hips.

8. Release and repeat on the other side by lifting your left leg and crossing it over your right thigh with your left arm under your right. Hold for fifteen seconds.

9. Repeat this five times on each side.

**Tips:**

You can start with your legs only and work on your focus and form before moving onto your arms.

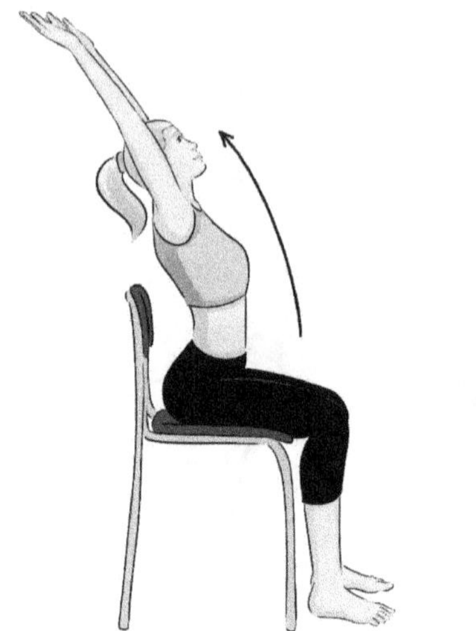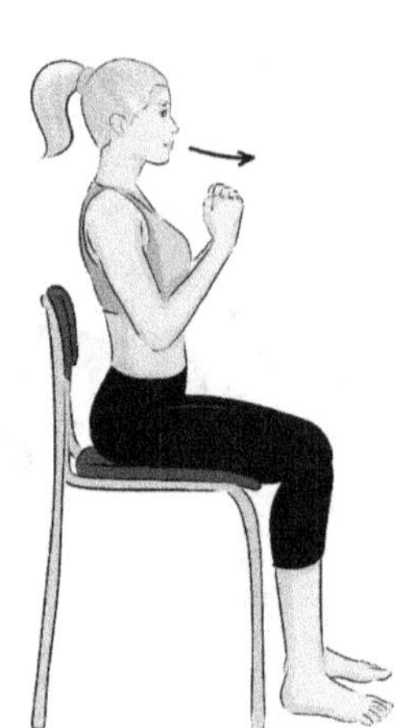

1. Sit on a chair with your feet flat on the ground and your back straight.

2. Interlace your fingers and take three deep breaths.

3. Extend your arms upward and backward with your palms open, lengthening your spine. Gently arch your back and look up if it's comfortable for your neck.

4. Hold this stretch for fifteen seconds.

5. Return to an upright, seated position with fingers crossed and take three deep breaths.

6. Repeat this three times, focusing on your breath and maintaining good posture.

**Tips:**

Remember your breathwork from the first few chapters? This is a great movement to practice the relaxing breath (the 4-7-8 technique).

## Heel Raises

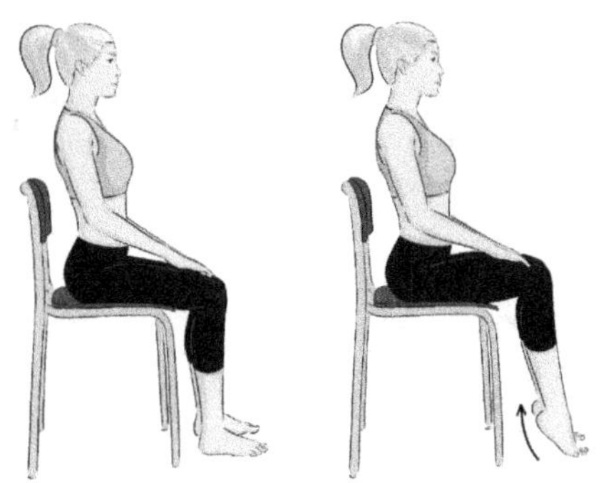

1. Sit on a chair with your feet flat on the floor and your back straight.

2. Place your hands on your thighs for stability.

3. Slowly lift your heels off the ground, raising them as high as you comfortably can.

4. Hold the raised position for a second or two.

5. Lower your heels back to the floor.

6. Repeat this motion fifteen times or up to twenty at a level that's comfortable for you.

**Tips:**

Remember to keep your back straight.

## Floor Leg Raise

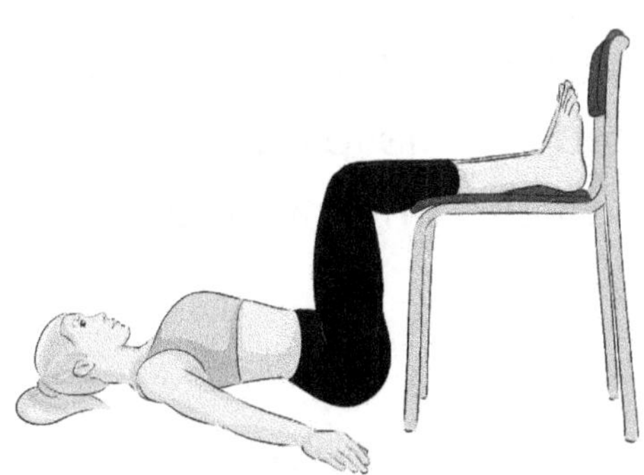

1. Lie down on a mat or the floor with your legs at a 90-degree angle on the chair.

2. Place your arms at your sides, palms facing up.

3. Relax and breathe deeply, holding the pose for thirty seconds. Sometimes, I stay here for up to a minute.

**Tips:**

You can raise your hands to the sides fully extended like a cross. This is also found in the Egoscue method. It realigns the hips and legs.

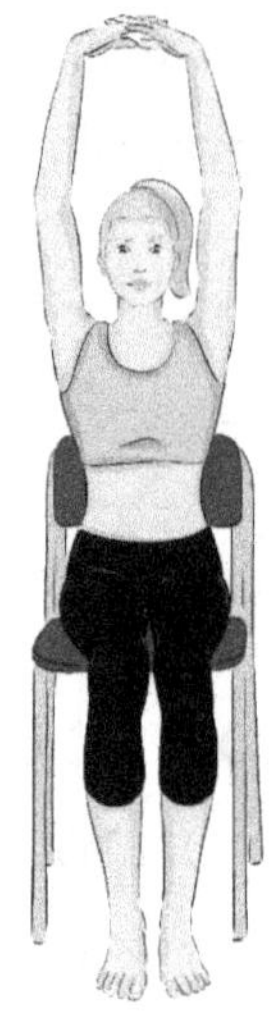 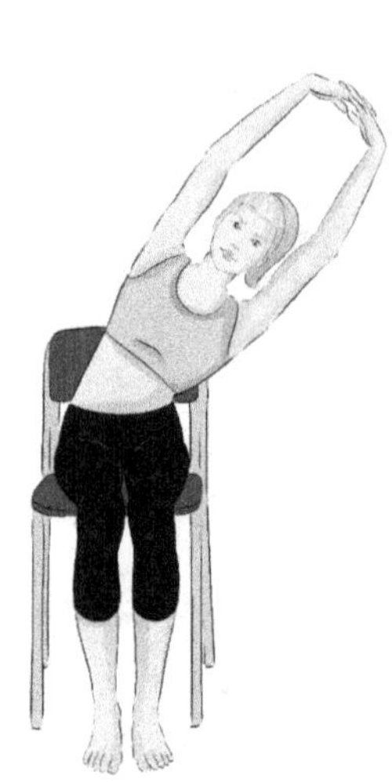

1 Sit on a chair with your back straight and your feet flat on the floor.

2 Inhale deeply as you extend both arms overhead, reaching for the sky.

3 Keep your palms facing upward and your fingers extended. Stretch your entire upper body, lengthening your spine. Feel the stretch from your fingertips to your shoulders.

4 Now move your arms to the right for five seconds; hold here, and take two deep breaths.

5 Now repeat on the left side.

6 To exit, gently lower your arms back to your thighs.

**Tips:**

- Remember to keep your head looking forward and your spine straight.

- You can repeat the stretch as needed to relieve upper body tension and improve posture while seated.

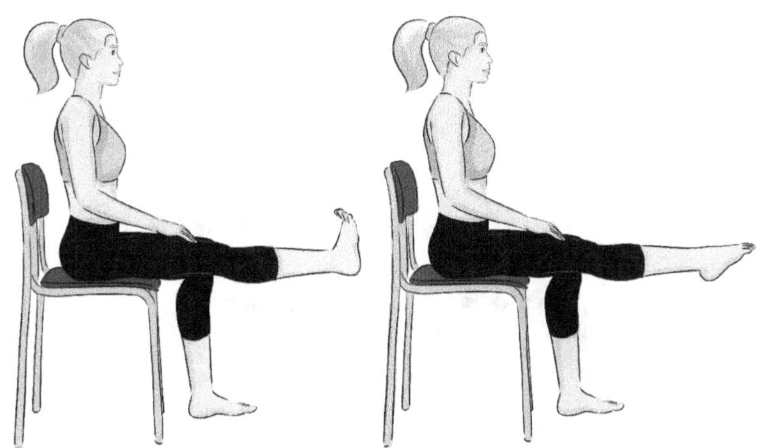

1 Sit on a chair with your back straight and your feet flat on the floor.

2 Engage your core muscles to stabilize your body.

3 Slowly lift one leg straight out in front of you with your toes pointed upward. Now, point them forward parallel to the floor.

4 Gently lower your leg back to the floor.

5 Repeat the motion five times.

6 Repeat the leg raise on the other side.

**Tips:**

You can place your hands on the sides of the chair or hold the armrests for support.

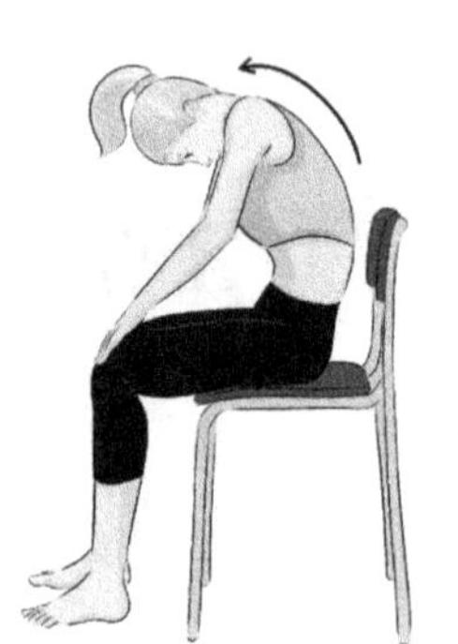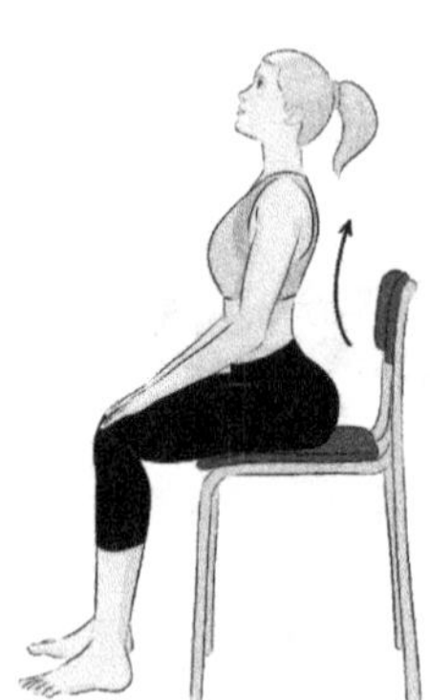

1. Sit on a chair with your feet flat on the floor and your back straight.

2. Place your hands on your knees or thighs.

3. Inhale and arch your back, lifting your chest (cow pose).

4. As you exhale, round your back, tuck your chin to your chest, and draw your navel in (cat pose).

5. Continue to flow between cow and cat poses with your breath, inhaling for the cow and exhaling for the cat.

6. Perform this gentle movement for ten reps, feeling the stretch and release in your spine.

**Tips:**

- You can place your hands on the sides of the chair or hold the armrests for support.

- Keep your movements smooth and controlled, focusing on your breath and the sensations in your back.

# Hand Stretch

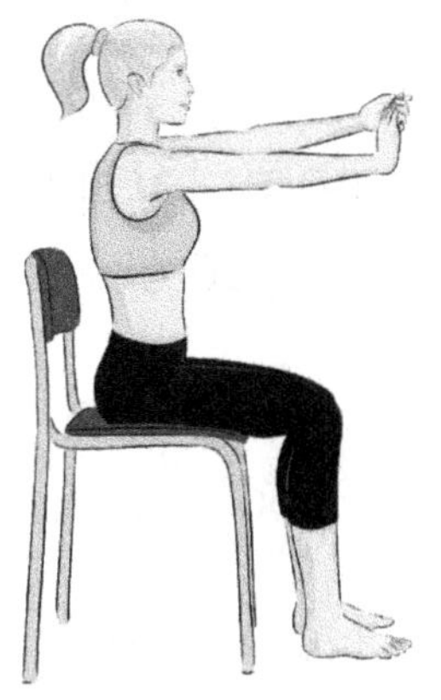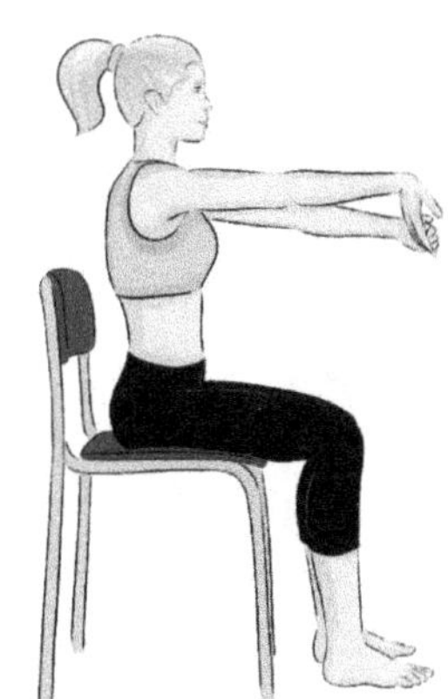

1. Sit or stand with your back straight.

2. Extend your right arm in front of you at shoulder height, palm facing outward.

3. With your left hand, gently grasp your right fingers or thumb.

4. Apply gentle pressure to stretch your fingers back toward your body.

5. Hold the stretch for fifteen seconds, feeling a gentle pull in your hand and fingers.

6. Switch to your left hand and repeat the stretch.

7. You can also stretch your fingers individually by gently pulling them backward.

**Tips:**

- Perform the stretch as needed to relieve hand tension and improve hand flexibility.

- You can do this anytime, even while standing up.

- Keep your head facing forward and your spine aligned when doing this.

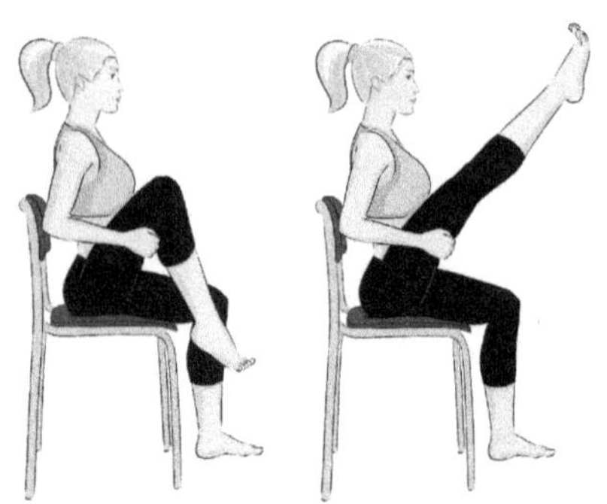

1  Sit on a chair with your feet flat on the floor, your back straight, and your hands on your thighs for stability.

2  Place both hands below one of your thighs and lift your thigh.

3  Now extend your feet upward. It's okay if you can't extend your leg completely straight. Just go as far as you comfortably can.

4  Release your leg and return to position 2 (both hands below the thigh).

5  Do seven reps.

6  Now repeat for the other leg.

**Tips:**

Try to keep your toes straight when your feet are off the floor.

## Seated Knee Stretch

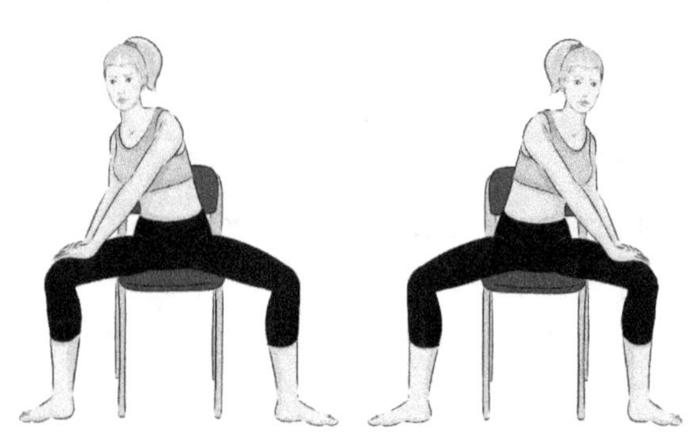

1  Sit comfortably on the chair and spread your legs as much as possible.

2  Place both hands on one knee and lean slightly forward. The turn comes from the torso, not the hips.

3  Hold for three seconds.

4  Now, turn and hold the other knee with your hands. Hold for three seconds.

5  Repeat this for a total of five times on each knee.

**Tips:**

Keep your head up and your spine aligned. Gain length by extending, not tightening, muscles

# Chair Half Warrior Pose

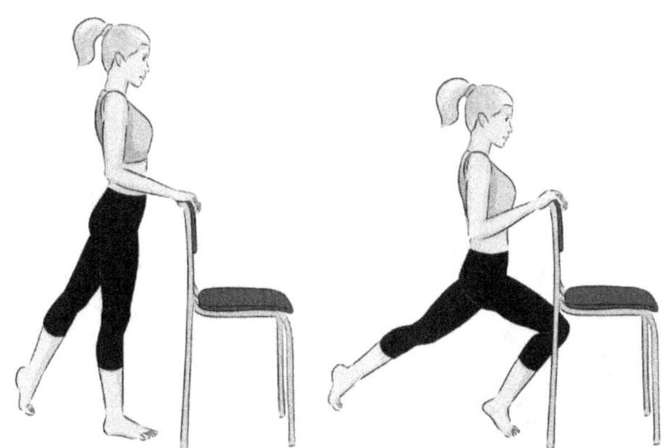

1. Begin in a standing position behind the chair.

2. Step your left foot back about three to four feet. As you do, bend your right knee and extend your left leg backward as far as you comfortably can.

3. Hold here for ten seconds. You can even push a little bit to see if you can go further. Use the chair for stability so you can push harder and further.

4. To exit the pose, step your back foot forward to the starting position.

5. Repeat the pose on the other side by stepping your right foot back and bending your left knee.

6. Repeat this exercise five times on each side.

**Tips:**

- As you gain more balance, you can put the chair to the side just in case you lose balance.

- You can also extend your arms toward the front and the back as in a normal warrior pose.

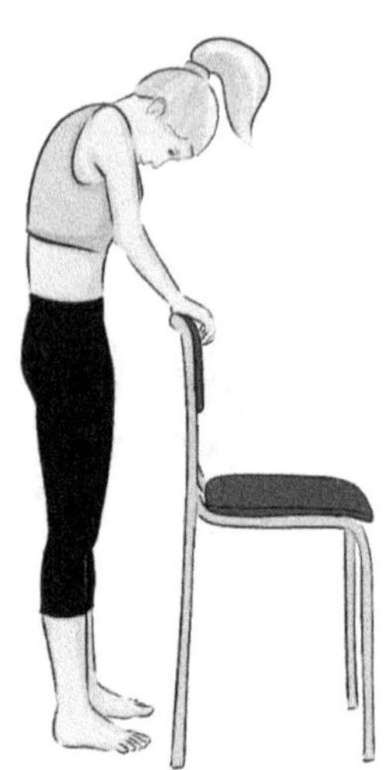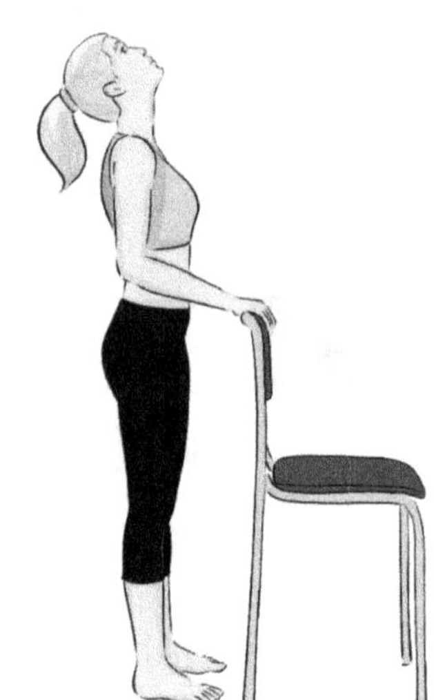

1. Stand with your back straight and your shoulders relaxed. Put your hands on the back of the chair for support.

2. Inhale deeply and, as you exhale, tilt your head downward, bringing your chin toward your chest. Hold for five seconds.

3. Now, raise your head upward and backward. Hold for five seconds.

4. Perform the downward and upward stretch for eight reps.

**Tips:**

- You can repeat this stretch as needed to relieve tension in your neck and shoulders. I do ten reps each morning.

- Keep your feet on the ground and your legs straight. A slight bend on the knees is fine.

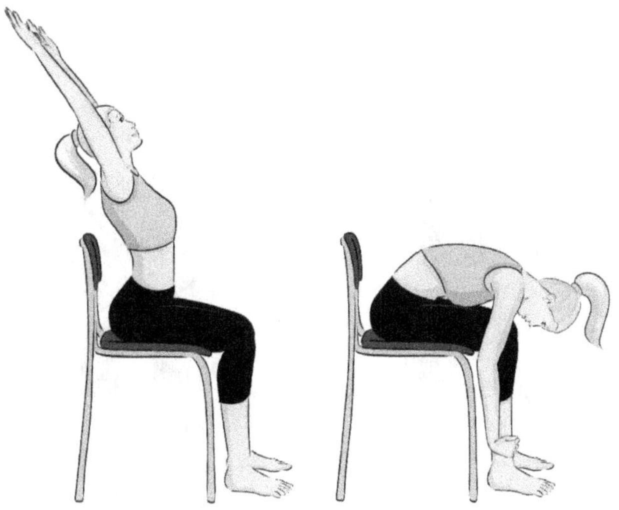

1. Sit on a chair with your back straight, your feet flat on the ground, and your hands resting on your thighs.

2. Inhale deeply and, as you exhale, raise your arms above and behind your head, reaching for the ceiling.

3. Hold the stretch for ten seconds, breathing deeply and evenly.

4. Now lean forward, bringing your chest to your knees, and go as deep as you can. Hold for ten seconds.

5. Repeat the above eight times.

**Tips:**

- You can hold your ankles when you go downward for stability.

- You can repeat both upward and downward stretches as needed to relieve tension and promote flexibility while sitting.

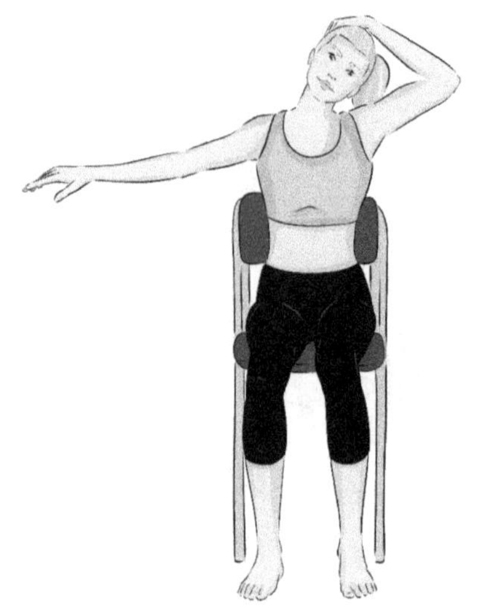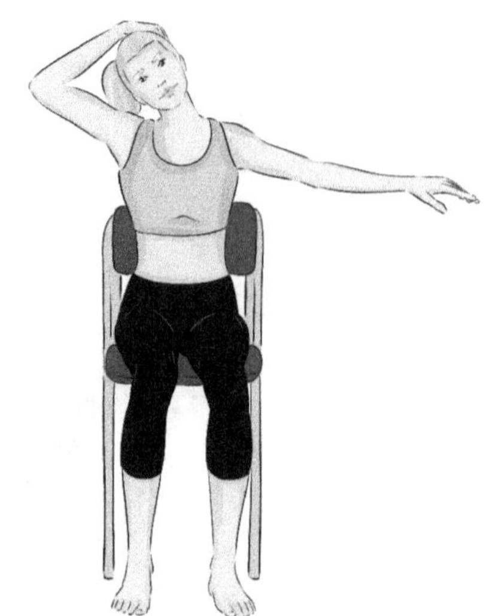

1. Sit on a chair with your feet flat on the ground and your back straight.

2. Place your right hand on your left ear and gently guide your head to the right, bringing your right ear toward your right shoulder.

3. Hold the head tilt for ten to fifteen seconds, feeling a gentle stretch along the left side of your neck.

4. Release your head and return it to an upright position.

5. Repeat this for the other side.

6. Perform these stretches as needed to relieve neck and arm tension and improve flexibility. I do five stretches each on the left and right side for a total of ten reps.

**Tips:**

- Be careful not to use too much force with your hand moving your head. Only go as far as comfortable.

- If you feel any pain at all, stop immediately. Some people have tension around the sternocleidomastoid (SCM) muscle and the levator scapulae muscle. In this case, consider releasing the trigger points first.

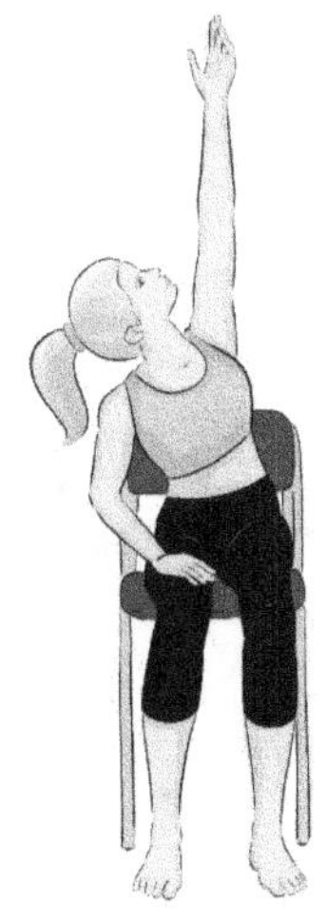 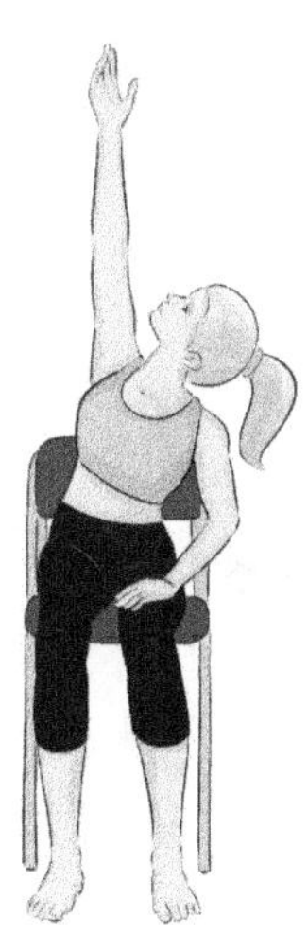

1. Sit on the chair with your legs in front of you.

2. Place your right hand on your lap. Inhale and lift your left arm overhead, stretching it toward the right side.

3. Exhale and extend your left hand upward.

4. Hold the pose for ten seconds, feeling a stretch along your left side.

5. Inhale and return to an upright seated position.

6. Repeat the stretch on the other side, placing your left hand on your lap and reaching your right arm overhead.

7. Perform these stretches as needed to improve flexibility and balance. I do five reps on each side for a total of ten.

**Tips:**

You can extend your resting hand toward the floor instead of your lap for a deeper stretch.

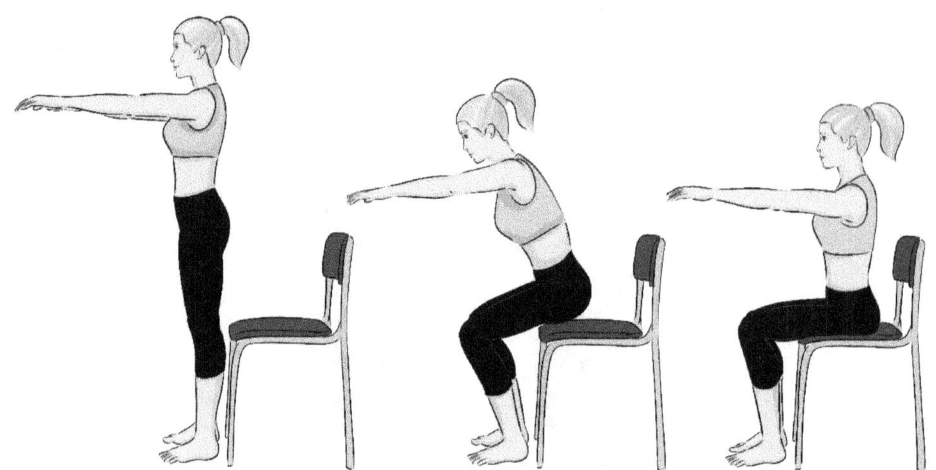

1. Sit on the edge of a sturdy chair with your feet flat on the ground, hip-width apart. Keep your back straight, your shoulders relaxed, and your arms by your sides.

2. As you exhale and engage your leg muscles, lift your hips off the chair.

3. Use your leg muscles to push through your heels to rise to a standing position. Hold the standing position for three seconds, ensuring your knees are not locked.

4. On your exhale, gently lower yourself back down to the chair.

5. Repeat the chair squat ten times, maintaining a controlled and smooth motion.

6. Focus on your breath and keep your core engaged to maintain balance.

**Tips:**

Think of your spine as aligned at all times as you move from a sitting to a standing position. Remember your posture training in exercises 1–3 and the Alexander technique.

# Next Steps

**_"Take care of your body. It's the only place you have to live."_**
*— Jim Rohn*

Once you get into the habit of these movements, you won't want to stop. Use the 28-Day Challenge program to stay motivated and on track. After a while... doing regular chair yoga exercises will make you feel more flexible, stronger, toned, and more vibrant in every way. After about eight weeks, this will become a habit for the rest of your life.

I know that some of you will want to continue on to more advanced exercises, so before we say goodbye, let me direct you to our exclusive free book on pelvic floor Kegels exercise at wallpilates.org as taught by Tim Sawyer, a leading physical therapist who worked with Dr. Anderson and Dr. Wise at the Stanford University Medical Center[*].

You can also check out our other exercise books here on Amazon.

You can also scan the following to get your free bonus:

---

[*]    Authors of *A Headache in the Pelvis: A New Understanding and Treatment for Chronic Pelvic Pain Syndromes*.

# Thank You

My name is Luna, and it has been my pleasure to serve you.

You could have picked from dozens of other books, but you took a chance and chose this one. So, thank you for investing in yourself and making it to the end!

Before we say goodbye, one question: If you enjoyed this book, would you consider leaving a review? A review is the easiest and best way to support the work of independent authors like me. Your feedback will help us continue writing the types of books that will help you and others in the journey to good health.

### How to leave a review in fifteen seconds:

Review This Chair Yoga Book

As you work on these exercises, by the fifth or sixth session, you will start to feel more aligned in your posture and feel like you're standing taller.

By the tenth session, you won't want to stop.

By the twentieth session, it will become a habit.

If you haven't started yet, what are you waiting for? Try out these movements for yourself and feel the truth in your body.


To your happiness and health,

— *Luna Light*

# Additional Resources

Use this URL from the National Pilates Certification Program to find a certified Pilates instructor:

https://nationalpilatescertificationprogram.org/NPCP/NPCP/Directory/CertifiedTeachersList.aspx

Find and add a certified yoga instructor search/association

# Disclosures

Some of the links provided in this book are affiliate links, which help you jump to the exact URL of the resource you're looking for at no additional cost to you.

# The Legal Stuff

**Assumption of Risk:** By reading/using this book, the User/Reader acknowledges that physical exercise involves inherent risks and hazards. By choosing to follow or participate in any exercise regimen, instruction, or advice detailed in the Book, the User expressly and voluntarily assumes all risks associated with such activities, recognizing that they may result in injury, illness, death, and/or damage to personal property.

**Waiver:** By reading this Book/Guide, the User hereby waives, releases, and forever discharges the author, publisher, and all related parties from any and all claims, liabilities, actions, suits, demands, costs, losses, damages, attorney's fees, and expenses, whether known or unknown, foreseen or unforeseen, that arise out of or relate to the User's/Reader's use of or reliance on the Book/Workout Guide.